MEDICAL BOARDS STEP 2
MADE RIDICULOUSLY SIMPLE

Andreas Carl, M.D., Ph.D.
Adjunct Assistant Professor
University of Nevada Reno
School of Medicine
Dept. of Physiology and Cell Biology
Reno, NV 89557-0046

MedMaster, Inc., Miami

D0110188

Notice: The author and publisher of this book have taken care to make certain that the recommendations for patient management and use of drugs are correct and compatible with the standards generally accepted at the time of publication. As new information becomes available, changes in treatment and use of drugs are inevitable. The reader is advised to carefully consult the instructions and information material included in the package insert of each drug or therapeutic agent before administration. The author and publisher disclaim any liability, loss, injury or damage incurred as a consequence, directly or indirectly, of the use and application of any of the contents of this book.

Diagnostic descriptions and criteria of psychiatric diseases have been adapted from the *Diagnostics and Statistical Manual of Mental Disorders*, Fourth edition (DSM IV) with permission of the American Psychiatric Association.

Copyright © 1997 by MedMaster, Inc.

All rights reserved. This book is protected by copyright. No part of it may be reproduced, stored in a retrieval system, or transmitted in any form or by any means, electronic, mechanical, photocopying, recording or otherwise, without written permission from the copyright owner.

ISBN # 0-940780-28-3

Made in the United States of America

Published by
MedMaster, Inc.
P.O. Box 640028
Miami, FL 33164

For Manfred, Rosi, Olaf and Astrid

In medical practice you will encounter uncommon presentations of common diseases.

On the Medical Board Exams you will encounter common presentations of uncommon diseases.

WHY SHOULD I BUY THIS BOOK ?

This book is not meant as a "Mini-Harrison" of Medicine. *Medical Boards Step 2 Made Ridiculously Simple* has only one single purpose: It is meant as a "**last minute review**" so that you will have the key facts required to pass the USMLE Step 2 exam ready at hand.

I have written it in a way to help you in the **decision making process**. For example, rather than listing all possible signs and symptoms of pulmonary embolism, you will find how to distinguish pulmonary embolism from myocardial infarction in a clinical setting. This has been accomplished by listing only the most important and most specific items in a table format, allowing you to rapidly compare similar or easily confused diagnoses. I believe that this approach will be most helpful both in multiple choice situations and when seeing real patients.

Most chapters of *Medical Boards Step 2 Made Ridiculously Simple* have two parts. A **Differential Diagnostics** section presented in table format and a **Hot-List** covering patient management of diseases listed by the National Board of Medical Examiners. You will find that many items on the USMLE Step 2 give patient data (history, symptoms and lab data) followed by the question "*what is the next most appropriate step in patient management?*" The hot-list of each chapter addresses just this question - what to do next ?!

While some may view the separation of diagnosis and management as somewhat artificial, I believe that it will make it easier for you to learn the essentials in the shortest possible time. Also keep in mind that diagnosis and management are different physician tasks and that you will actually receive two separate scores for these on your USMLE Step 2 exam.

iv

Additional parts of this book are: a list of **Signs and Symptoms** and an overview of commonly used **Diagnostic Tests** including their indications and interpretations. Since you are not required to know specific surgical techniques, I have included surgical topics along with the other disciplines.

How you score on the USMLE Step 2 exam not only depends on how hard you study, but also on what you study. Obviously, if you study what they ask, you will achieve a very high score. I have prepared this manuscript in order to help you maximize your efforts. The material has been selected based on my experience with medical exams in Germany and my more recent experiences with the USMLE Step 1 and USMLE Step 2 exams in the United States.

I have tried to write the book I wish I would have had when I studied for the USMLE Step 2 exam and I have included all the information I wish I would have known when I took this exam.

I like to thank Dr. Suat Yasar and Dr. Bouke de Jong for their numerous helpful suggestions and critical reading of this manuscript, Dr. Stephen Goldberg for his editorial help and Steve Goldberg for providing his lively illustrations.

Good luck, and please let me know any comments or suggestions you may have for future editions.

Thanks !

STUDY HINTS

There are three areas from the USMLE Step 1 which you will need to know:

- **Pathology** - disease entities and mechanisms of disease
- **Microbiology** - infectious diseases
- **Pharmacology** - drug indications, side effects and contraindications

These topics are covered in detail in my book *Medical Boards Step 1 Made Ridiculously Simple*. In order to avoid repetition and to keep the present book as compact as possible I have not repeated this information here. I strongly advise you to spend at least one day each reviewing these areas.

BOOKS / MULTIPLE CHOICE QUESTIONS

Many excellent books are on the market, and you should have no difficulty choosing the right one for your personal learning style. It is usually better to know one book really well than to know a little of many books. I prefer the medium size text books, for example *"Cecil Essentials of Medicine"* (1) or *"Rudolph's Fundamentals of Pediatrics"* (17) over the somewhat shorter "pure review books" (Oklahoma Notes or NMS series). The extra material will improve your understanding and medical judgment and they are easier to read too.

You should practice at least a few hundred multiple choice questions under "real time" conditions before the actual exam. I particularly recommend the *National Medical Series Review for the USMLE Step 2* (14). These are most similar in style and difficulty to the real exam. Mark all the ones you got wrong and concentrate your studies on these areas. I made myself "error sheets" listing all my mistakes in single line statements. The day before the exam I read this list of facts I should have known to give me a last minute extra boost. It worked !

MEDICINE

The current political emphasis on primary care and family practice is reflected in the content of the USMLE Step 2. You would be very well advised to use any of the primary care medicine books for your preparation. **I especially recommend *"Medicine: A Primary Care Approach"*** (13). If you have somewhat limited time and want to read only one book - this is it. It is divided into 127 short chapters dealing with the common medical problems, each preceded by a case history. Great new book !

PREVENTIVE MEDICINE / PUBLIC HEALTH

This often underestimated topic is a very important part of the Medical Boards. You should know the risk factors of most cancers and leading causes of death. You should know immunization schedules for both children and adults. You should know when to do screening tests, and when not to do screening tests.

SURGERY

No knowledge of any special surgical techniques is required - but you should know the difference between a Billroth-I and Billroth-II. Learn all you can about automobile accidents, the different types of injuries (blunt versus perforating trauma) associated with them and their treatment. It's a favorite topic.

OB/GYN

High yield topics: Normal development (puberty and menopause), menstrual cycle, infertility, differential diagnosis of bleeding during pregnancy, management of medical complications during pregnancy. Try to memorize major drugs that are contraindicated during pregnancy, and those which are allowed. *Obstetrics and Gynecology* by W.W. Beck (15) is my favorite from the NMS series - an easy to digest book covering the essentials.

PEDIATRICS

Despite what they say about children not being "little adults", there is significant overlap with internal medicine. If you choose to read a full book like *"Rudolph's Fundamentals of Pediatrics"* (17) you may want to concentrate on just a few chapters like neonatology, congenital defects, transmission of STDs during pregnancy and/or labor, nutrition, normal development and endocrine diseases.

PSYCHIATRY

Really all you need to know are the diagnostic definitions published in *"Quick Reference Guide to the DSM IV"* (16). If you have difficulty applying these somewhat abstract concepts to real cases you may want to read a few chapters in the *"DSM IV - Casebook"* (7). Remember: Biological psychiatry and drug treatment is "in." Psychoanalysis is "out."

TEST TAKING STRATEGIES

Many questions are extraordinarily long. I recommend to read the last sentence of a long question first, then take a quick glance at the answers. This way you know what they want before you endeavor to work your way through the patient's history and lab-data.

If you can't even guess a question, choose either the longest answer or the one that is most similar to other choices. Then move on. Watch your time - it's critical !

ADVICE FOR FOREIGN MEDICAL GRADUATES

In contrast to your American peers you should take this exam very seriously. With the recent changes in health care policy it has become more and more difficult to find residency positions. Your score on the USMLE Step 2 may very well determine what kind of residency position you will get or if you "get in" at all. Your goal should not be to "just pass it," but to achieve an above average score (200 or better) and you should prepare yourself accordingly.

- Practice as many multiple choice questions as you can and practice at least a few hundred under real time conditions (stop watch).

- Learn patient management as well as possible, especially if you are from a country where health care delivery and the spectrum of diseases differ from the US.

- Work through the cases in *Internal Medicine Pearls* (11).

- If you can, take advantage of morning or noon conferences at your local University Hospital.

REFERENCES

1. Cecil Essentials of Medicine, W.B. Saunders Co.
2. Cecil Textbook of Medicine, W.B. Saunders Co.
3. Current Medical Diagnosis&Treatment, Appleton&Lange
4. Current Emergency Diagnosis&Treatment, Appleton&Lange
5. Current Obstetric&Gynecologic Diagnosis&Treatment, Appleton&Lange
6. Current Pediatric Diagnosis&Treatment, Appleton&Lange
7. Diagnostics and Statistical Manual of Mental Disorders, American Psychiatric Press
8. DSM IV Casebook, American Psychiatric Press
9. Harrison's Principles of Internal Medicine, McGraw-Hill
10. Internal Medicine, Ed. J.H. Stein, Mosby
11. Internal Medicine Pearls, Mosby-Yearbook
12. Mayo Internal Medicine Board Review, Mayo Foundation
13. Medicine: A Primary Care Approach, W.B. Saunders Co.
14. National Medical Series Review for the USMLE Step 2, Williams&Wilkins
15. Obstetrics and Gynecology, NMS series, Harwal Publishing
16. Quick Reference to the Diagnostic Criteria from DSM IV, Am. Psychiatric Press
17. Rudolph's Fundamentals of Pediatrics, Appleton&Lange
18. Rudolph's Pediatrics, Appleton&Lange
19. Synopsis of Psychiatry, Williams&Wilkins

WORLD-WIDE-WEB SUPPORT

- latest trends on USMLE
- new updates
- hot links
- If you just took this exam and wish to share your experience, your thoughts would be much appreciated!

www.med.unr.edu/homepage/andreas

CONTENTS

TABLE OF CONTENTS

PUBLIC HEALTH ISSUES

SIGNS AND SYMPTOMS

DIAGNOSTIC TESTS

PEDIATRICS

INJURY AND POISONING

NEUROLOGY

PSYCHIATRY

PUBLIC HEALTH ISSUES

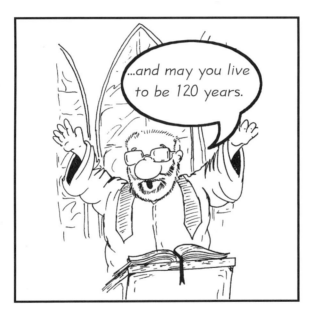

The leading cause of death in people age 120...
curses.

Part A : Epidemiology

1.1.) <u>POPULATION DATA</u>

birth rate	live births / population
fertility rate	live births / females age 15 to 45
death rate	deaths / population
miscarriage	fetal death within first 20 weeks
stillbirth	fetal death at 28 weeks or later
neonatal mortality rate	deaths (<28 days) / live births
perinatal mortality rate	stillbirths + deaths (< 7 days) / total births
infant mortality rate	deaths (<1 year) / live births
maternal mortality rate	pregnancy-related deaths / live births

 Rates are reported per 1000 population per year except maternal mortality per 100,000 per year.

1.2.) <u>LEADING CAUSES OF DEATH</u>

neonates	**- prematurity** - congenital abnormalities
infants	**- congenital abnormalities** - injuries
teenagers, young adults	**- motor vehicle accidents** [1] **- homicide** - suicide
adults > 40 years	**- heart disease** - lung cancer - cerebrovascular disease
elderly	**- heart disease** - cerebrovascular disease - lung disease
death due to drug overdose	- tricyclic antidepressants

 [1] *Homicide is the leading cause of death in black teenagers.*
Suicide and accidents are more common in white teenagers.

1.3.) <u>SEX</u>

male	female
- coronary artery disease - cardiomyopathy	- mitral valve prolapse
- endangitis obliterans - periarteritis nodosa	- Raynaud's phenomenon
- alcoholic cirrhosis - hemochromatosis	- primary biliary cirrhosis
- ankylosing spondylitis - Reiter's syndrome	- lupus erythematodes - scleroderma - arthrosis of finger joints
- COPD, lung carcinoma etc.	- endocrine diseases
- gout - porphyria - chronic lymphocytic leukemia - hairy cell leukemia	- anorexia nervosa

1.4.) ETHNICITY

Caucasians	- cystic fibrosis
Mediterraneans	- β-thalassemia - G6PD deficiency
African Americans	- hemoglobinopathies (HbS, HbC) - α-thalassemia, β-thalassemia - G6PD deficiency - hypertension - homicide
Eskimos	- pseudocholinesterase deficiency
Ashkenazi Jews	- Gaucher's - Niemann-Pick - Tay-Sachs

1.5.) <u>OCCUPATION</u>

abattoir workers	- brucellosis
bakery	- flour, fungi, dust (asthma)
battery manufacture or repair	- lead poisoning - cadmium poisoning
cotton industry	- byssinosis
dentists	- mercury
farmers	- pesticides - actinomycosis - brucellosis - erysipeloid - alveolitis
gardeners	- sporotrichiosis
glass and ceramics industry	- silicosis, lead poisoning
insulation industry **ship building**	- asbestosis - mesothelioma
mining	- dust, coal, silica
painters	- solvents - lead poisoning
radiator repair	- lead poisoning
rubber industry	- aromatic amines (bladder carcinoma)

1.6.) <u>GEOGRAPHY</u>

coccidioidomycosis	- Southwestern United States
histoplasmosis	- Ohio/Mississippi river
Lyme disease	- East Coast and Midwest of USA - Scandinavia
Rocky Mountain spotted fever	- East Coast of the USA (not Rocky Mountains !)
Western equine encephalitis	- West of Mississippi
Eastern equine encephalitis	- Atlantic and Gulf states
California encephalitis	- North-Central States of USA

1.7.) <u>ANIMALS</u>

pasteurella	- cat bites, dog bites
anthrax	- cattle, swine, wool
brucellosis	- cattle (dairy products) - goats (dairy products) - pigs
hanta virus	- deer mice
toxoplasmosis	- cat feces
psittacosis	- birds
leptospirosis	- rats, dogs, cats
Rocky Mountain spotted fever (Rickettsia rickettsii)	- dogs, rodents -> ticks -> humans
epidemic typhus (Rickettsia prowazekii)	- humans -> lice -> humans
endemic typhus (Rickettsia typhi)	- rodents -> fleas -> humans
tularemia	- rabbits -> ticks -> humans
Lyme disease (Borrelia burgdorferi)	- mice -> ticks -> humans
plague (Yersinia pestis)	- squirrels, rats
Chagas' disease (Trypanosoma)	- kissing bug
kala-azar (Leishmania)	- sandfly

1.8.) <u>RISK AND ODDS</u>

	disease present	disease absent
risk factor present	A	B
risk factor absent	C	D

- ***risk***   : $A / (A+B)$
- ***odds***   : A / B

- ***risk ratio*** : $[A / (A+B)] / [C / (C+D)]$
- ***odds ratio*** : $[A / B] / [C / D]$

- ***attributable risk***   : $\text{risk}_{exposed} - \text{risk}_{unexposed}$
- ***relative risk (risk ratio)*** : $\text{risk}_{exposed} / \text{risk}_{unexposed}$

If risk is small (A << B), risk and odds will be almost the same

---

  - **Risk ratio** can be determined from prospective **cohort study**.
  - Risk ratio <u>can not</u> be determined from case-control study.

  - **Odds ratio** can be determined from **case-control study**.
  - If risk is low, odds ratio will give a good estimate of risk ratio.

Type I error: To say there is a difference between groups when there is not (α).
Type II error: To say there is no difference between groups when there is (β).

Power : $1 - \beta$

Part B : Preventive Medicine

1.9.) TYPES OF PREVENTION

primary prevention	- predisease - vaccinations - prevention of nutritional deficiencies - prevention of specific injuries
secondary prevention	- latent disease - early detection of disease - screening
tertiary prevention	- symptomatic disease - limitation of physical and social consequences of disease - rehabilitation

1.10.) <u>CORONARY HEART DISEASE</u>

<u>Risk Factors</u> :

fixed	modifiable
- male sex	- cigarette smoking
- family history	- high LDL
- older age	- low HDL
	- diabetes mellitus
	- hypertension

Cessation of smoking decreases most excess risk within 1 year.

<u>Reducing risk factors:</u>
- slows progression of coronary disease.
- may even result in a slight regression in some patients.
- significantly reduces coronary events.

1.11.) <u>PULMONARY DISEASE</u>

	examples
primary prevention	- avoid environmental exposure - avoid occupational exposure - stop smoking
secondary prevention	**- PPD screening** indications: - close contacts of persons with tuberculosis - immigrants from Africa, Asia, South America - residents of nursing homes etc. - HIV positive persons
tertiary prevention	**- COPD:** - monitor blood oxygen saturation - supplemental oxygen prolongs life

 *Screening otherwise asymptomatic cigarette smokers for lung cancer (e.g. chest x-ray or sputum cytology) does not improve overall survival and is **not recommended**.*

1.12.) <u>OSTEOPOROSIS</u>

bone formation	bone loss
- estrogen - testosterone - calcium - vit. D	- glucocorticoids - parathyroid hormone - thyroid hormone
- weight bearing exercise	- renal failure

type I	type II
- **"postmenopausal"** - affects only women	- **"senile"** - affects men and women

- develops rapidly
- loss of trabecular bone
  (vertebrae, forearm)
	- develops more gradually
	- trabecular and cortical bone
	  (femoral neck, tibia, pelvis)

- bone loss is most rapid during first 5 years post menopause.
- bone loss resumes if estrogen replacement is discontinued.
- up to 30% of bone is lost before detectable by x-ray.
- DEXA scan preferred over CT or photon absorptiometry.

- testosterone may be useful for men with gonadal deficiency.

1.13.) <u>PREGNANCY SCREENING</u>

hypertension	- monitor throughout pregnancy (weight gain, edema, blood pressure)
Rh incompatibility	- determine at first prenatal visit
rubella titer	- determine at first prenatal visit
STDs	<u>at first prenatal visit:</u> - gonorrhea - syphilis - chlamydia - HBsAg - offer HIV
bacteriuria	- urine culture at first prenatal visit - treat bacteriuria, even if asymptomatic
triple screen [1]	- at 16-18 weeks
oral glucose tolerance	- at 24-28 weeks
amniocentesis	- consider for women > 35

[1] α-FP , hCG , estriol

1.14.) <u>NEONATAL SCREENING</u>

phenylketonuria	- all infants at birth
hypothyroidism	- all infants at birth
hemoglobin electrophoresis	- African - Mediterranean - South East Asian

1.15.) <u>RHESUS FACTOR</u>

- **if unsensitized Rh- mother with Rh+ (or unknown) father:**
  give immunoglobulins at 25-30 weeks gestation.

- **if unsensitized Rh- mother delivers Rh+ infant:**
  give second dose of immunoglobulins within 72 hours after delivery.

1.16.) <u>IMMUNIZATIONS FOR INFANTS</u>

	birth	2m	4m	6m	15m	4-6y
hepatitis B	●	●		●		
hemophilus influenzae		●	●	●	●	
oral polio		●	●		●	●
DTP, DTaP		●	●	●	◐	◐
MMR					●	●

 If mother positive for HBsAg also give immunoglobulins to newborn.

Oral Polio (Sabin):	*- live-attenuated*
	- lifelong immunity
	- local gut and systemic immunity
	- may cause paralytic disease
Injectable Polio (Salk):	*- inactivated*
	- requires booster every 4-5 years
	- minimal gut immunity
	- no risk of paralytic disease

16

1.17.) <u>IMMUNIZATIONS FOR ADULTS</u>

dT	- every 10 years
measles	- if born before 1957 : assume "natural" immunity - if born after 1957 : recommend 2 doses - protective if given within 72 h of exposure - pregnant or immune compromised : give IgG
pneumovax **(give once)**	- elderly > 65 years - chronic ill persons: COPD, HIV, CHF, DM etc. - prior to splenectomy
influenza **(every autumn)**	- elderly > 65 years - chronic ill persons: COPD, HIV, CHF, DM etc. - contacts and health care personnel

 No live vaccines for HIV positive infants or adults <u>except MMR</u> !

1.18.) IMMUNIZATION REACTIONS

if present:	avoid:
allergy to egg	- MMR - influenza
allergy to neomycin	- MMR - oral polio
immunodeficiency	- MMR (but is o.k. for HIV+ patients) - oral polio
neurologic disorder	- DTP

1.19.) <u>TETANUS PROPHYLAXIS</u>

	tetanus toxoid	tetanus immune globulin
3 or more doses		
- clean minor wound	yes if > 10 years	no
- other wound	yes if > 5 years	no
immunization unknown or less than 3 doses		
- clean minor wound	yes	no
- other wound	yes	yes

1.20.) CANCER RISK

lung cancer	- smoking - secondhand smoke - radiation (radon)
nasopharyngeal cancer	- smoking - alcohol
cervix cancer	- early age at first intercourse - multiple sex partners
breast cancer	- no or late pregnancies - obesity - high fat diet - radiation (mammography ?)
liver cancer	- hepatitis B or C infection - vinyl chloride
colon/rectum cancer	- diet high in saturated fat - diet low in fruits, vegetable, fiber
bladder cancer	- aromatic amines
skin cancer	- sun light (UV-B radiation)

Cigarette smoking also increases the risk of:
- *cervix cancer*
- *bladder cancer*
- *pancreas cancer*

1.21.) <u>CANCER SCREENING</u>

breast cancer	> 40 years : annual clinical exam > 50 years : **mammography** every 1-2 years
cervix cancer	- Pap smears every 1-3 years - for all women who are or have been **sexually active**
prostate cancer	> 40 years : **digital rectal exam** - routine PSA screening not recommended
colon cancer	- fecal occult blood if > 50 years or family history - **colonoscopy if family history of polyposis**
testicular cancer	- if history of **cryptorchidism or testicular atrophy**
ovarian cancer	- routine screening **not recommended**
endometrial c.	- routine screening **not recommended** - watch for abnormal uterine bleeding in elderly women
lung cancer	- routine screening **not recommended**

1.22.) <u>SOCIAL INSURANCE</u>

MEDICARE	MEDICAID
- part of Social Security Trust Fund	- paid from general tax revenue
- federally administered	- administered by the States
- for people > 65 years - for people who receive social security benefits due to disability	- for poor people (usually on welfare)

- covers some home care
- covers some nursing home care
- covers most but not all hospitalization
	- pays medical care expenses
	- pays long-term nursing home care
	  after personal resources have been
	  exhausted

Part C : Drug Abuse

1.23.) ABUSE & DEPENDENCE

abuse	dependence
recurrent substance use resulting in:	recurrent substance use resulting in:
- failure to fulfill obligations - dangerous situations (e.g. DUI) - social difficulties - legal difficulties	- **tolerance*** - **withdrawal syndromes*** - unsuccessful efforts to quit - preoccupation with obtaining drug resulting in loss of social, occupational or recreational activities.

* indicates physiological dependence

 - *Almost all drugs can cause delirium during intoxication.*

- *Withdrawal delirium is only common with alcohol, sedatives and anxiolytic drugs.*

1.24.) <u>ALCOHOL AND SEDATIVES</u>

intoxication	withdrawal

- slurred speech
- unsteady gait
- incoordination
- nystagmus
	"uncomplicated" [1]
	6-8 hours after cessation
	  - autonomic hyperactivity
	  - seizures
	  - hand tremor
	  - insomnia
	  - nausea, vomiting
	
	perceptual disturbances
	8-12 hours after cessation
	  - delusions, hallucinations
	
	delirium tremens
	72 hours after cessation
	  - agitation, unpredictable behavior
	  - lost reality testing
	  - mortality 20% if untreated

[1] even uncomplicated (i.e. no delirium) withdrawal may be life threatening !

<u>Perceptual disturbance:</u>
Hallucinations and illusions with <u>intact reality testing</u>, i.e. the patient knows that these are due to drug rather than external reality.

<u>Drug-induced Psychotic Disorder:</u>
Hallucinations and Illusions with <u>lost reality testing</u>.

1.25.) CANNABIS

intoxication	withdrawal
- euphoria - anxiety - sensation of slowed time - social withdrawal - **conjunctival injection** - dry mouth - increased appetite	- none

1.26.) LSD

intoxication	withdrawal
- marked anxiety - paranoid ideas - fear of losing one's mind - pupillary dilation - tachycardia - sweating - tremors	- none **flashbacks**: reexperiencing hallucinations and illusions after cessation of drug use

1.27.) <u>AMPHETAMINES / COCAINE</u>

intoxication	withdrawal
- euphoria - vigilance - anxiety, tension - **pupillary dilation** - tachycardia or bradycardia - psychomotor agitation or retardation - weight loss	- dysphoria - fatigue - unpleasant dreams

1.28.) OPIOIDS

intoxication	withdrawal
- initial euphoria - then apathy - **pupillary constriction** - slurred speech - drowsiness, coma	- **severe, but not life threatening** - dysphoria - nausea, vomiting, diarrhea - sweating, lacrimation - muscle aches, fever

1.29.) PHENCYCLIDINE

intoxication	withdrawal

- aggressive, impulsive behavior
- agitation
 	
- **horizontal and vertical nystagmus**
- hypertension
- ataxia
- muscle rigidity
- hyperacusis
- seizures
	- none, but psychosis may last
	  for days or weeks following
	  use of PCP

SIGNS AND SYMPTOMS

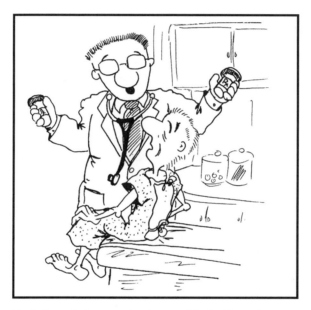

"The first drug is to control your high blood pressure.
The second drug is to counteract the *first drug's* side effects,
but can have its own side effect of *increasing* the blood
pressure. But not to worry. If that happens, simply take
more of the first medicine."

2.1.) <u>CARDIOVASCULAR SIGNS</u>

S3 gallop (ventricular)	**- dilated cardiomyopathy** - *may be normal in children and young adults* - aortic insufficiency - congestive heart failure - volume overload
S4 gallop (atrial)	**- constrictive cardiomyopathy** (stiff ventricle) - *may be normal in athletes* - arterial hypertension - myocardial ischemia or infarction - AV block
pulsus paradoxus	**- exaggerated decline of BP during inspiration** - cardiac tamponade - constrictive pericarditis - massive pulmonary embolism
pulsus alternans	**- beat to beat change in pulse amplitude** - indicates left ventricular failure
orthopnea	**- difficulty breathing in supine position** (increased hydrostatic pressure in pulmonary circulation) - COPD - left ventricular failure
Kussmaul's sign	**- distention of jugular veins with inspiration** - constrictive pericarditis

2.2) <u>RESPIRATORY SIGNS</u>

Biot	- breaths of equal volume alternating with episodes of apnea - a/w central cerebral lesions
Cheyne Stokes	- **waxing and waning** (hyperpnea <-> apnea) - common at high altitude - a/w increased intracranial pressure
Kussmaul	- hyperventilation (**deep, rapid, sighing**) - a/w metabolic acidosis
barrel chest	- **increased ant./post. diameter** of chest - late sign of COPD - due to loss of lung elasticity
breath odors	- **fruity**: ketoacidosis - **sweet, musty**: liver failure - **uriniferous**: uremia, renal failure - **foul**: lung abscess, bronchiectasis
nasal flaring	- **respiratory distress** - important sign in children who can't tell !

2.3.) <u>AUSCULTATION</u>

crackles (rales, crepitations)	- rattling noises, usually during inspiration - movement of air through fluid-filled airways - **bronchitis, pneumonia, lung edema**
rhonchi	- continuous, resembles deep snore - narrowing of large airways - **aspiration, bronchospasm**
wheezing	- rhonchi with high-pitched musical quality - cannot be cleared by coughing - **bronchospasm, mucosal edema, asthma**

stridor	- loud, musical sound
	- usually inspiratory
	  (may be expiratory in severe cases)
	
	- **obstruction of larynx or trachea**
	- may indicate life threatening narrowing of
	  airways, especially in children

2.4.) EYES AND EARS

scotoma	**areas of partial blindness** - glaucoma - chorioretinitis - macular degeneration - migraine (scintillating scotomas)
arcus senilis	- green-white, opaque ring at corneal periphery - fat deposits
Horner's syndrome	**damage to cervical chain ganglia** resulting in: - pupil constriction - ptosis (eye lid drooping) - warm, dry facial skin
hearing loss	**conductive hearing loss** [1] - cerumen - tympanic membrane perforation - otitis media - otosclerosis **sensorineural hearing loss** [2] - presbyacusis - ototoxic drugs - Méniére's - acoustic neurinoma
tinnitus	**ear ringing** - acoustic neurinoma - labyrinthitis - Méniére's disease - small tympanic membrane perforations - hypertension - **salicylates, quinine, aminoglycosides**

[1] Weber lateralizes towards sick ear.
[2] Weber lateralizes towards healthy ear.

2.5.) <u>INFECTIONS</u>

Brudzinski's sign	**- meningeal irritation** - flexion of hips and knees in response to passive flexion of neck
Kernig's sign	**- meningeal irritation** - hamstring muscle pain when examiner lifts the supine patient's extended leg
opisthotonus	**- meningeal irritation** - severe muscle spasm causing back arch - more common in infants
McBurney's sign	**- appendicitis** - rebound tenderness at McBurney's point (1/3 from ant. sup. spine to umbilicus)
Murphy's sign	**- acute cholecystitis** - arrest of inspiration when palpating liver
Koplik's spots	**- measles** - small red spots with bluish-white center on buccal mucosa - generalized rash will follow in 1-2 days
Janeway spots [1]	**- infective endocarditis** - tiny red lesions on palms and soles
Roth spots [1]	**- infective endocarditis** - subretinal hemorrhages with pale center
Osler's nodes [1]	**- infective endocarditis** - tender, raised nodules on finger pads and toes

[1] these "famous signs" are actually not very common.

2.6.) <u>RHEUMATIC DISEASES</u>

Heberden's nodes	**- osteoarthritis** - painless bony enlargement of DIP
swan neck deformity	**- rheumatoid arthritis** - hyperextended PIP - slightly flexed DIP also: - volar subluxation of MCP - ulnar deviation of fingers
tophi	**- gout** - painless, nodular swelling (uric acid deposits) - ears, hands, feet

2.7.) <u>MALIGNANCIES</u>

Virchow's node	- palpable supraclavicular lymph node - a/w stomach cancer
Pancoast's	- shoulder pain (brachial plexus) - Horner's syndrome (cervical chain ganglia) - a/w apical lung tumors
Lambert-Eaton	- myasthenia - a/w small cell carcinoma (lung)
Trousseau's	- migratory thrombophlebitis - a/w adenocarcinomas: breast, lung, prostate...
peau d'orange	- edematous thickening of breast skin - a/w breast cancer (late sign)

2.8.) <u>TRAUMA</u>

Battle's sign [1]	**- basilar skull fracture** - ecchymosis over mastoid - develops 24-36h after trauma
Racoon's eyes [1]	**- basilar skull fracture** - bilateral periorbital ecchymosis
Cullen's sign	- indicates **intraabdominal bleeding** - hemorrhagic patches around umbilicus
Turner's sign	**- intraabdominal bleeding** - hemorrhagic patches at flanks
anterior drawer sign	- anterior cruciate ligament
posterior drawer sign	- posterior cruciate ligament
McMurray's sign	**- meniscal tear** - "click" or "pop" elicited by lower leg manipulation

[1] important since basilar skull fractures are easily missed on x-ray.

2.9.) <u>MISCELLANEOUS</u>

carpopedal spasm	**tetany, hypocalcemia**
Trousseau's sign **Chvostec's sign**	- carpopedal spasm induced by inflating cuff on upper arm for several minutes - spasm of facial muscles elicited by tapping the patient's lower jaw area just anterior to earlobe
Homan's sign	- deep calf pain resulting from dorsiflexion of foot - indicates **deep venous thrombosis**
Nicoladoni's sign	- bradycardia when applying pressure to **arteriovenous fistula**
Ortolani's sign	- "click" upon abduction of a newborn's thigh. - indicates **congenital hip dysplasia**
Rumpel-Leede sign	- place a tourniquet around upper arm and watch for distal petechiae - indicates severe **thrombocytopenia**
spider angioma	- a form of telangiectasia - most common on face and neck - characteristic for **liver cirrhosis**
pica	**- craving for inedible substances** - in children may indicate malnutrition, iron deficiency… - in adults usually indicates psychological disturbance

2.10.) <u>NERVE & MUSCLE</u>

asterixis	- "flapping tremor" - most commonly involves **wrist joint** and fingers - hallmark of hepatic encephalopathy - also seen in uremic syndrome
ataxia	- **incoordination of voluntary movements** - cerebellar - sensory (impaired proprioception)

athetosis	- **slow involuntary snakelike** movements
	  (especially face, neck and upper extremities)
	- due to damage of basal ganglia,
	  e.g. birth hypoxia, kernicterus
	- often combined with chorea

chorea	- bursts of **rapid, jerky movements** - may appear purposeful - **Huntington's**: chorea plus intellectual decline - **Wilson's** disease: chorea plus hemolytic anemia - sometimes caused by phenothiazines
cogwheel rigidity	- **jerking of arm muscles when passively stretched** - cardinal sign of Parkinson's - sometimes caused by antipsychotic drugs
dysdiadochokinesia	- **difficulty performing rapidly alternating movements** - cerebellar disease
Gower's sign	- sign of **proximal muscle** weakness (Duchenne, Becker) - characteristic maneuver to rise from the floor
fasciculations	- minor muscle contractions (single motor units) **do not cause joint movements** - normal in tense, anxious or tired persons - early sign of organophosphate poisoning

2.11.) <u>REFLEXES</u>

sucking reflex **palmar grasp reflex**	- weak in premature infants - fully developed after 36 weeks of gestation

tonic neck reflex	- turn face to one side (supine position):
	  arms and leg on face side will extend
	
	 - indicates neurological dysfunction if
	  constantly present

Babinski reflex	- firmly stroke lateral sole of feet - dorsiflexion of great toe, fanning of other toes **- normal up to 2 years of age**
Moro reflex	- "startle reflex" - flexion of leg - embracing posture of arms **- normal up to 6 months of age**

automatic walking	- full-term newborns at 40 weeks tend to
	  "walk" in heel-toe progression
	
	 - preterm infants at 40 weeks tend to "walk"
	  in toe-heel progression

 An asymmetric Moro reflex occurs with Erb's palsy (birth trauma).

2.12.) <u>BRAIN STEM</u>

doll's eye sign	- indicates **brain stem dysfunction when absent** (i.e. eyes remain fixed in midposition when head is turned from side to side) - absent doll's eye is normal in neonates - don't do when cervical spine injury is suspected !
Argyll Robertson pupils	- small, irregular pupils - **respond to near accommodation** - **do not respond to light** - syphilis stage 3 (tabes dorsalis)
decorticate posture	- **legs extended, arms flexed** - damage to corticospinal tract - better prognosis than decerebrate
decerebrate posture	- **legs and arms extended** - damage to upper brainstem

2.13.) <u>PSYCHIATRIC SIGNS</u>

aphasia	receptive[1] or expressive[2] language disorder
apraxia	failure to do, despite intact motor function
agnosia	failure to recognize
dementia	- gradual impairment of cognitive functions, memory - **Alzheimer** : early memory loss - **multi-infarct** : steplike decline
delirium	- **acute, organic, short lasting** - clouded consciousness - confusion, disorientation, anxiety - sometimes hallucinations
delusions	- persistent false belief despite invalidating evidence - grandeur - paranoia - somatic delusions
illusions	- misperception of external stimuli
hallucinations	- perception without external stimuli

---

[1] ***Wernicke:*** *- speech is fluent but rambling*
- patient has difficulty understanding spoken or written language

[2] ***Broca:*** *- word-finding difficulty resulting in non-fluent speech*
- little or no difficulty understanding spoken or written language

---

 Both Wernicke's and Broca's patients cannot repeat words or phrases.

DIAGNOSTIC TESTS

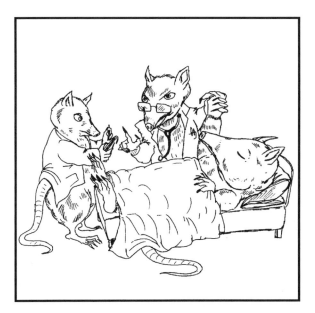

"Just drop his hand over his head. He doesn't want
to hurt himself. If it hits his head, he's comatose.
If it misses, he's playing possum."

3.1.) <u>WATER AND SALT</u>

hyponatremia **high osmolarity**	- **hyperglycemia** - use of hypertonic mannitol
hyponatremia **normal osmolarity**	- **hyperlipidemia** - **hyperproteinemia** (e.g. multiple myeloma)
hyponatremia **low osmolarity**	- **SIADH** - renal failure
hypernatremia [1] **ECV expanded**	- indicates **net Na$^+$ gain** - if mild: Cushing's or hyperaldosteronism - if severe: patient who received hypertonic saline
hypernatremia [1] **ECV depleted**	- **diarrhea, sweating, renal losses** - if patient is not thirsty, suspect hypothalamic tumor

[1] always a/w hyperosmolarity !

- *Evaluate plasma Na$^+$ always in the context of osmolarity and ECV.*

- *Correct hypernatremia and hyponatremia very slowly (0.5 mM/hour).*
  (danger of central pontine myelinolysis !)

3.2.) <u>POTASSIUM AND CALCIUM</u>

hypokalemia	**- Hyperaldosteronism**
	  - Conn (low renin)
	  - Bartter (high renin)
	
	- loss
	  - renal (diuretics)
	  - diarrhea
	  - laxative abuse
	
	- transcellular shift: **alkalosis**
	               acute glucose load
	               insulin excess

hyperkalemia	**- Addison's** **- ACE inhibitors** - artifact: RBC hemolysis during blood drawing - rhabdomyolysis, tumor lysis - distal renal tubular acidosis - transcellular shift: **acidosis**
hypocalcemia	**- chronic renal failure** (phosphate retention) - lack of dietary Ca^{2+} and vit. D - hypoparathyroidism
hypercalcemia	**- bone cancer**, metastases - hyperparathyroidism - hypervitaminosis D

Free Ca^{2+} depends on pH :
acidosis -> high free Ca^{2+}
alkalosis -> low free Ca^{2+} (tetany)

3.3.) pH AND BLOOD GAS

simple hypoxia (Pa_{CO_2} normal)	- ARDS - pneumonia
respiratory acidosis	- pH < 7.35; Pa_{CO_2} > 45 mmHg - COPD
metabolic acidosis	- pH < 7.35; HCO_3 < 24 mmEq/l - **check anion gap !** - ketoacidosis - renal failure - acute MI
respiratory alkalosis	- pH > 7.45; Pa_{CO_2} < 35 mmHg - anxiety, hysteria - pulmonary embolism - salicylate intoxication (early phase)
metabolic alkalosis	- pH > 7.45; HCO_3 > 28 mmEq/l - severe vomiting - gastric suction - hypokalemia

---

Anion gap = $[Na^+]$ - $[Cl^- + HCO_3^-]$ = 8-12 mM/l

Normal anion gap   - *diarrhea*
                                         - *renal tubular acidosis*

Increased anion gap   - *lactic acidosis*
                                         - *ketoacidosis*
                                       - *salicylates*
                                       - *alcohol (ethanol etc.)*

3.4.) <u>LIVER & KIDNEYS</u>

AST (GOT)	- **hepatitis** - **acute MI** : detectable: 6-10 h peak: 24-48h - **drugs**: antibiotics, oral contraceptives...
gamma-GT	- persistent liver cell damage - **alcoholism** - **drugs**: aminoglycosides, warfarin...
bilirubin	- **direct (conjugated):** - biliary obstruction - drug induced cholestasis - Dubin-Johnson, Rotor's - **indirect (unconjugated):** - hemolytic anemia - physiologic jaundice of the newborn - Gilbert's, Crigler-Naijar...
BUN	- **renal failure** - dehydration - high protein intake
creatinine [1]	- **renal failure** - **diet** (meat...)

uric acid	- **gout**
	- **leukemia, metastatic cancer**
	  chemotherapy !
	- **food high in purines:**
	  brain, heart, kidneys, roe, sardines, scallops

[1] **creatinine clearance** is more sensitive indicator of renal function (GFR)

3.5.) <u>BLOOD LIPIDS</u>

cholesterol	**TC = HDL + LDL + VLDL** **= HDL + LDL + triglycerides/5** TC > 240 mg/dl : increased risk for CHD LDL > 160 mg/dl : increased risk for CHD HDL < 35 mg/dl : increased risk for CHD HDL > 60 mg/dl : considered "protective" LDL/HDL < 4 desirable
triglycerides	- increased levels with age - TG > 200 mg/dl : increased risk for CHD - estrogen and oral contraceptives increase triglycerides

> ***Rule out secondary causes of hyperlipidemia:***
> - *diet: alcohol, saturated fats*
> - *drugs: steroids, thiazides, beta-blockers*
> - *diseases: diabetes, hypothyroidism, uremia*

3.6.) <u>IRON</u>

serum iron	**increase** : hemolysis hemochromatosis hemosiderosis **decrease** : anemia of chronic disease iron deficiency anemia blood loss
ferritin	**increase** : hemochromatosis hemosiderosis **decrease** : iron deficiency anemia
total iron binding capacity (transferrin)	**increase** : blood loss iron deficiency anemia oral contraceptives ! **decrease** : anemia of chronic disease cirrhosis nephrotic syndrome
transferrin saturation	- **if < 15%** : iron deficiency anemia

3.7.) <u>ELECTROPHORESIS</u>

A) SERUM

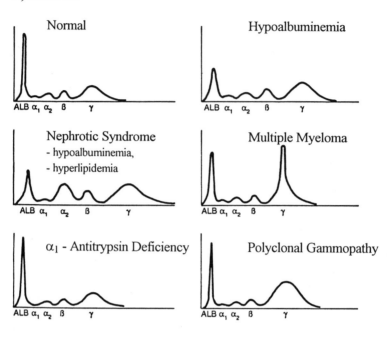

B) URINE

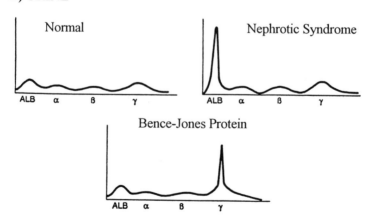

From *Clinician's Pocket Reference,* 8th edition, page 75, edited by L.G. Gomella.
Appleton & Lange, 1997. Used with permission.

3.8.) IMAGING - 1

chest x-ray (CXR)	- pneumonia - pneumonitis - neoplasms, metastases - no routine screening for lung cancer !
expiratory CXR	- to visualize small pneumothorax
lateral decubitus CXR	- to visualize small pleural effusions
lung V/Q scan	- normal scan rules out pulmonary embolism
pulmonary angiography	- most accurate diagnostic procedure for embolism, but do only if V/Q scan is "non-diagnostic" - AV malformation
acute abdominal series (for initial evaluation)	- supine and upright, abdominal and CXR - watch for gas pattern, foreign bodies, renal and liver shadows, psoas shadow
barium enema	- indications: unresolved diarrhea, heme-pos. stools, change in bowel habits
air-contrast barium enema	- double contrast delineates mucosa - polyps, ulcerative colitis
ERCP	- visualizes common bile and pancreatic ducts - stones, obstructions, ductal pattern - may induce acute pancreatitis !

3.9.) IMAGING - 2

ultrasound	- **B mode**: two-dimensional, fetal imaging - **M mode**: measurement of cardiac chambers and movement of all 4 valves - **Doppler**: to quantitate blood flow
IV pyelogram	**pyelonephritis** - small kidneys - deformed calyces **glomerulonephritis** - kidneys and calyces look normal **polycystic kidney** - large kidney - "spider" calyces
retrograde pyelogram	- if kidneys and ureters could not be visualized on IV pyelogram - can be done if patient is allergic to IV contrast
^{99m}Tc sulfur colloid scan	- detects GI bleeding
hepatobiliary scintigram	- ^{99m}Tc IDA - nonvisualization of gall bladder is diagnostic for obstruction of cystic duct (acute cholecystitis)
thallium scan	- myocardial perfusion - normal myocardium appears "hot" - **ischemic areas appear "cold"**
^{99m}TC pyrophosphate scan	- **recently damaged myocardium appears "hot"**

3.10.) __TOMOGRAPHY__

MRI	CT
MRI is better than CT for:	**CT is better than MRI for:**
- brain, spinal cord - soft tissues - renal masses	- subdural/epidural hematomas
Disadvantages:	**Disadvantages:**
- claustrophobia - longer scanning time - contraindicated if patient has metallic implants / pacemakers	- radiation exposure

3.11.) CLASSIC X-RAY SIGNS

Kerley's B lines	- congestive heart failure - lung edema
unilateral high diaphragm	- paralysis - atelectasis - abscess
coin lesions (lung)	- calcified granulomas - primary carcinoma - metastases
egg-shell calcifications (hilar lymph nodes)	silicosis, sarcoidosis
ground glass appearance	- sarcoidosis, miliary tbc - pneumoconiosis
honeycombing	- endstage lung fibrosis
water bottle	- pericardial effusion
beak-like	- esophagus achalasia
lead-pipe	- ulcerative colitis
cobble-stoning	- Crohn's disease
napkin-ring	- colon cancer (right side)
apple core	- colon cancer (left side)
cotton-wool skull	- Paget's disease
punched out radiolucent areas of skull	- multiple myeloma

CARDIOVASCULAR DISEASES

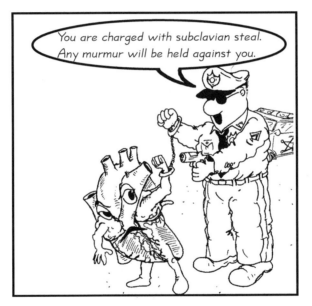

Cardiac arrest.

301 - 277 - 0617

4.1.) ECG PATTTERNS: ELECTROLYTES

hypokalemia	**- prolonged, flat T waves** - U waves	mild severe
hyperkalemia	**- tall, peaked T waves** - widening of QRS	mild severe
hypocalcemia	**- prolonged ST segment**	
hypercalcemia	- shortened ST segment	
digitalis	**- prolonged PR interval** (watch for AV block) **- shortened QT interval** - (watch for ectopic systoles) **- deep, scooped ST**	

4.2.) <u>ECG PATTERNS : ISCHEMIA</u>

q waves	- transmural infarction
ST depression	- subendocardial ischemia
ST elevation	- transmural ischemia - coronary artery spasm
T wave inversion	- nonspecific finding - may be present after MI - transient T wave inversion during ischemia

 A normal ECG does not exclude coronary artery disease or acute MI.

<u>Q waves, ST elevations, T inversions :</u>

	in leads :		arteries :
anteroseptal	V1 - V3	I, aVL	LAD
anterolateral	V4-V6	I, aVL	CRFLX
inferior		II, III, aVF	RCA
posterior	reciprocal V1 - V3		RCA

4.3.) <u>ECG PATTERNS : ARRHYTHMIAS</u>

sick sinus	- paroxysmal tachycardias / bradycardias - normal p waves, normal QRS
AV block - 1 degree	- PR interval > 0.2 s
AV block - 2 degree	- **Mobitz type I (Wenckebach)** - progressive lengthening of PR interval followed by QRS dropout
AV block - 2 degree	- **Mobitz type II** - constant PR, sudden dropouts of QRS - Adam-Stokes syncope
AV block - 3 degree (complete)	- P waves independent of QRS - QRS wide if originating in ventricle
Wolff-Parkinson-White	- accessory AV pathway causing pre- excitation - may trigger reentrant tachyarrhythmias - short PR interval < 0.12 s - increased QRS > 0.12 s - **delta waves** (= slurred QRS) : - a/w Ebstein's anomaly

4.4.) <u>PACEMAKERS</u>

not indicated	indicated
- asymptomatic sick sinus syndrome - asymptomatic atrial fibrillation	- symptomatic second degree AV block (Mobitz I)
- **first degree** AV block	- second degree block (Mobitz II) even if asymptomatic
- **asymptomatic second degree** AV block (Mobitz I)	- third degree AV block

59

4.5.) <u>CARDIAC ENZYMES</u>

CK (MB fraction)	most sensitive and specific marker of MI acute MI : **- detectable at 6-12 h** - peak at 12-20 h
LDH 1	acute MI : **- detectable at 12-24 h** - peak in 2-5 days **LDH 1 : cardiac, RBCs** LDH 2 : cardiac, RBCs LDH 3 : lung LDH 4 : liver, skeletal muscle, kidney LDH 5 : liver, skeletal muscle **LDH1 / LDH2 > 1 ("flipped") : indicates MI**

 Negative creatine kinase MB at admission does not rule out MI.

 20-30% of infarctions are "silent" (common in diabetic patients).

4.6.) CARDIAC CAUSES OF CHEST PAIN

classic angina	- substernal pain - transient (<10 min) - provoked by exercise - relieved by rest or nitrates - **ST depression**
unstable angina	- change in pattern (more frequent, severe or prolonged) - angina at rest or at night - **ST depression**
variant angina (Prinzmetal's)	- due to coronary artery vasospasm - not provoked by exercise ! - **ST elevation**
myocardial infarction	- substernal pain -> arm, shoulder, jaw - lasts > 30 min - not relieved by rest or nitrates - **ST elevations, T inversions**
pericarditis	- sharp chest pain - aggravated by deep breathing - pericardial friction rub - **non-specific ST elevations**
dissecting aortic aneurysm	- "tearing" knifelike pain - sudden onset, long duration - may radiate to neck, chest or back

__Contraindications for stress testing__:
- *recent onset of unstable angina*
- *uncontrolled hypertension*
- *severe congestive heart failure*

4.7.) <u>OTHER CAUSES OF CHEST PAIN</u>

pulmonary embolism	- sudden onset dyspnea / tachypnea - pleuritic chest pain - hemoptysis indicates pulmonary infarction
pneumothorax	- sudden onset sharp pain - aggravated by breathing - hyperresonant to percussion - absent tactile fremitus
pleurisy	- well localized pain - aggravated by breathing - dull to percussion
peptic ulcer	- burning, gnawing pain - lower substernal area, epigastrium - relieved by food or antacids
psychosomatic	- sharp, often localized to a point - usually of short duration

4.8.) COMPLICATIONS OF MI

arrhythmia	- dizziness, palpitations - syncope
congestive heart failure	- dyspnea, orthopnea - S3 gallop, S4 gallop - rales, wheezes (cardiac asthma) - cardiogenic shock
myocardial rupture	- tamponade, shock, death - typically occurs with **small infarcts** !
papillary muscle rupture	- hyperacute onset pulmonary edema - loud systolic murmur (mitral regurgitation)
septal rupture	- new onset holosystolic murmur
ventricular aneurysm	- reduced ejection fraction - mural thrombi -> arterial emboli
pericarditis	**- occurs 1-3 days after MI** - pleuritic pain, non-responsive to nitrates - diffuse ST elevations - self-limited
Dressler's syndrome	**- occurs several weeks after MI** - pericardial and pleural effusions - fever, joint pain - tends to recur

4.9.) <u>HEART VALVES</u>

mitral stenosis	- **diastolic opening snap** - **diastolic rumble** - **loud S1** - **no S3 or S4** - dyspnea, orthopnea - atrial fibrillation
mitral regurgitation	- **holosystolic murmur** - **may radiate to axilla** - **widely split S2 (early A2)** - pulmonary congestion
mitral valve prolapse	- **midsystolic click followed by murmur** - palpitations - atypical chest pain
aortic stenosis	- **harsh systolic ejection murmur** - **may radiate to carotids** - angina - exertional syncope
aortic regurgitation	- **diastolic decrescendo murmur** - "waterhammer pulse" - **DeMusset**: head bobbing - **Traube**: pistol shot sounds over arteries - **Quincke**: pulsatile blushing of nail beds

4.10.) <u>AUSCULTATORY TRICKS</u>

: *Inspiration: - increases venous return*
 - increases rightsided murmurs

	OCM	AS	MR
Valsalva (decreases venous return)	↑	↓	↓
squatting (increases systemic vasc. resist.) (increases venous return)	↓	↑	↑
amyl nitrate (decreases arterial pressure) (increases cardiac output)	↑	↑	↓

OCM: obstructive cardiomyopathy, **AS**: aortic stenosis, **MR** mitral regurgitation
↑ : increases murmur,   ↓ : decreases murmur

physiologic split	- **P closes after A** (inspiratory split)
wide split	- **P closes after A** (inspiratory >> expiratory) - pulmonary stenosis - mitral regurgitation - RBBB
paradoxical split	- **A closes after P** (expiratory split) - aortic stenosis - tricuspid regurgitation - LBBB
fixed split	- **split independent of respiration** - ASD, VSD

4.11.) <u>PERICARDITIS</u>

infectious	**- often preceded by "cold"** - Coxsackie A and B and ECHO virus - tuberculosis - AIDS : atypical mycobacteria
metabolic	**- uremia** large effusions tamponade **- myxedema** large effusions rarely tamponade
post MI	**- early** (1-3 days after MI) self-limited, common **- Dressler's** (weeks after MI) uncommon

 ECG shows generalized (= nonspecific) ST elevations.

<u>cardiac tamponade</u>:
- *elevated venous pressure*
- *venous pulse : no y-descent*
      (impaired cardiac filling)
- *pulsus paradoxus*
- *ECG : low voltage, alternans*

4.12.) <u>CARDIOMYOPATHY</u>

dilated (congestive)	**- dilated ventricle, normal wall thickness** **- left and right ventricular failure** - alcohol - doxorubicin - infections (mainly viral)
hypertrophic	**- ventricular hypertrophy** **- small cavity** **- septum may obstruct outflow** - often genetic
restrictive	**- low ventricular compliance** **(restricts diastolic filling)** - amyloidosis - sarcoidosis - hemochromatosis

4.13.) <u>HEART FAILURE</u>

left heart	right heart
- dyspnoea - orthopnea - wheezes (cardiac asthma) - S3 gallop - S4 gallop - pulsus alternans	- peripheral edema - nocturia - jugular vein distention - hepatomegaly - splenomegaly

4.14.) <u>FUNCTIONAL CLASSES</u>
(New York Heart Association)

Class I	- no limitation of physical activity
Class II	- ordinary physical activity causes symptoms
Class III	- less than ordinary physical activity causes symptoms
Class IV	- symptoms at rest

4.15.) <u>SHOCK</u>

cardiogenic	**- cool, pale skin** **- distended neck veins** - myocardial infarction - cardiomyopathy - arrythmias
hypovolemic	**- cool, pale skin** **- collapsed neck veins** - hemorrhage - diabetes - Addison's
septic	**- warm, dry skin** **- edema despite hypovolemia** (low peripheral resistance) [1] - gram negative infections (endotoxins)
anaphylactic	**- pruritus, urticaria** **- respiratory distress** - IgE mediated

[1] *prognosis worsens if septic shock converts to a hypovolemic shock (with high systemic resistance).*

4.16.) <u>PERIPHERAL VASCULAR DISEASES</u>

arteriosclerosis	- atheromas - large and medium vessels
thrombangitis obliterans (Buerger's disease)	- intima proliferation - medium and small vessels - common in smokers
arterial embolism	- sudden onset - painful - absent pulse - atrial fibrillation -> atrial thrombus
Raynaud's phenomenon	- vasospasm of finger arteries - cyanosis followed by hyperemia - precipitated by cold or emotional upset <u>causes</u> - cryoglobulins - cold agglutinins - connective tissue diseases - neurologic disorders
thrombophlebitis	- inflammation of veins - usually painful

phlebothrombosis [1]	- may be asymptomatic
	- deep vein phlebothrombosis -> emboli
	
	- **Virchow's triad** : - stasis
	                      - endothelial injury
	                      - hypercoagulability

 [1] ***Homan's sign*** : *Famous, but neither specific nor sensitive !*

4.17.) <u>AORTIC ANEURYSMS</u>

arteriosclerotic	dissecting
- often asymptomatic	- severe, sudden, tearing pain
- most commonly located in lower abdominal segment	- most commonly begins in ascending segment, then extend distally, proximally or in both directions
- pulsatile abdominal mass	- wide mediastinum on CXR

Marfan's syndrome	syphilis
- involves first portion of aorta -> aortic valve insufficiency	- ascending aorta - obliteration of vasa vasorum
- media necrosis	
- rupture is common cause of death in Marfan's syndrome	

Hot-List

HEART MUSCLE

Coronary Artery Disease
- aggressive risk factor modification: 1. stop smoking 2. control blood pressure 3. lower lipids aggressively 4. control of blood glucose in diabetic patients
- nitrates as needed. Hospitalize if two doses 5 min. apart do not improve angina
- aspirin unless contraindicated (bleeding diathesis etc.)

Myocardial Infarction
- pain relief (morphine)
- watch for ventricular arrhythmias (lidocaine prophylaxis ?)
- reperfusion (thrombolysis, coronary angioplasty) within 6 hours
- thrombolysis is relatively contraindicated if bleeding from other sites likely (recent surgery or trauma, oral anticoagulation, cerebrovascular disease etc.)
- systemic anticoagulation (contraindicated if postinfarction pericarditis present)
- β-blockers, aspirin

Hypertrophic Cardiomyopathy
- dilated heart: digitalis, diuretics
- hypertrophic heart: β-blockers
- diuretics (hypovolemia) and glycosides increase obstruction !

Heart Failure
- control excess salt and water: sodium restriction, diuretics
- reduce workload: vasodilators, intra-aortic balloon pump
- improve cardiac performance: digitalis

ARRHYTHMIAS

- "trial and error" drug therapy
- pacemaker indications see table 4.4

Supraventricular Tachyarrhythmias
- β-blockers
- adenosine

Atrial Flutter/Fibrillation
- digoxin, β-blockers, Ca-antagonists
- cardioversion if hypotension or heart failure develops

Ventricular Fibrillation
- cardioversion (300-400 J)
- lidocaine
- bretylium, amiodarone etc.

WPW
- quinidine to prolong AV time

ENDOCARDIUM AND VALVES

Rheumatic Fever
- penicillin
- continue prophylaxis for 5-10 years after acute episode
- continue prophylaxis indefinitely if risk of infection is high

Infective Endocarditis
- obtain blood cultures
- start antibiotics based on clinical setting: drug users (Staph. aureus), indolent course (Viridans streptococci) etc.
- all patients with aortic or mitral valve disease should receive prophylaxis (amoxicillin or erythromycin) if undergoing dental or other procedures.

Mitral Stenosis
- may be present for lifetime with few symptoms
- watch for atrial fibrillation ! Anticoagulation !
- if pulmonary edema develops: balloon valvuloplasty

Mitral Regurgitation
- if acute (rupture of chordae tendinae): emergency surgery
- balloon counter pulsation helps

Mitral Valve Prolapse
- usually benign
- watch for ventricular arrhythmias
- treat chest pain with β-blockers
- antibiotic prophylaxis is not necessary if "click" is the only symptom

Aortic Stenosis
- significant risk of sudden death: Avoid strenuous exercise.
- valve replacement if symptomatic
- in children and young adults: consider valve replacement even if asymptomatic to decrease risk of sudden death

Aortic Regurgitation
- timing of valve replacement is difficult: (not too early, not too late)
- monitor ventricular function: output, ejection fraction, end-diastolic pressure

PERICARDIUM

Pericarditis
- viral and post MI: NSAIDs. Short course of steroids if pain persists
- Dressler's: avoid steroids !
- bacterial: drainage and antibiotics
- uremia: diuresis, pericardectomy if necessary

Tamponade
- if patient stable: emergency echocardiogram (confirmative)
- if patient deteriorates rapidly: emergency thoracotomy

BLOOD VESSELS

Hypertension
- exclude secondary causes: renal disease, renovascular hypertension, Cushing's, aldosteronism etc.
- diet, exercise
- first line drugs: β-blockers (patients with exercise anginal pain)
                     diuretics (black patients)
- others: ACE inhibitors, calcium antagonists, α1-blockers, α2-agonists

Atherosclerosis
- control risk factors for coronary heart disease
- niacin for all hyperlipidemias except hyperchylomicronemia
- bile acid resins (cholestyramine etc.) for hypercholesterolemia
- fibrates lower VLDL: good for hypertriglyceridemia

Shock
- rapid volume restoration (blood, colloids, crystalloids)
- Swan-Ganz catheter to determine hemodynamics
- vasoactive drugs, e.g. dopamine, to maintain perfusion pressure
- if sepsis: immediate broad spectrum antibiotics

Arteritis
- most forms respond well to corticosteroids
- cytotoxic agents if necessary
- early therapy to prevent blindness in patients with temporal arteritis

Aortic Aneurysm
- surgery if diameter > 5 cm (increased risk of rupture !)

Aortic Dissection
- untreated: about 20% mortality within 24 h.
- if type I or II (involves ascending aorta): surgery
- if type III (descending aorta only): medical treatment o.k.
  (β-blockers and afterload reduction to stabilize dissection)

Thrombophlebitis
- heat and elevation
- antibiotics if caused by indwelling catheter
- low-dose subcutaneous heparin to prevent phlebothrombosis

Phlebothrombosis
- same as for thrombophlebitis plus anticoagulation
- streptokinase only for serious ileofemoral phlebothrombosis
- if recurrent or anticoagulation is contraindicated: consider vena cava umbrella

RESPIRATORY
DISEASES

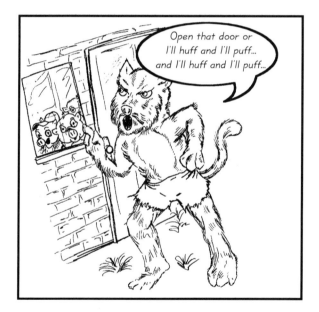

Emphysema in wolves.

5.1.) <u>PULMONARY FUNCTION TESTS</u>

vital capacity	VC = ERV + IC **- decreased in COPD**
residual volume	RV = TLC - VC **- increased in obstructive disease** **- normal or decreased in restrictive disease**
FVC, FEV$_1$	- most important parameters to monitor in asthma and pre-operative screening

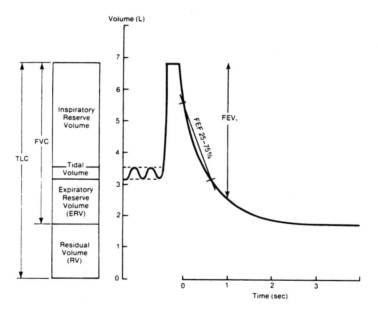

From *The Merck Manual of Diagnosis and Therapy*, 16th edition, p. 609, edited by R. Berkow.
Copyright 1992 by Merck & Co., Inc., Rahway, NJ. Used with permission.

5.2.) <u>FLOW VOLUME LOOPS</u>

A) Normal

B) Restrictive

D) Obstructive

C) Upper Airway Obstruction

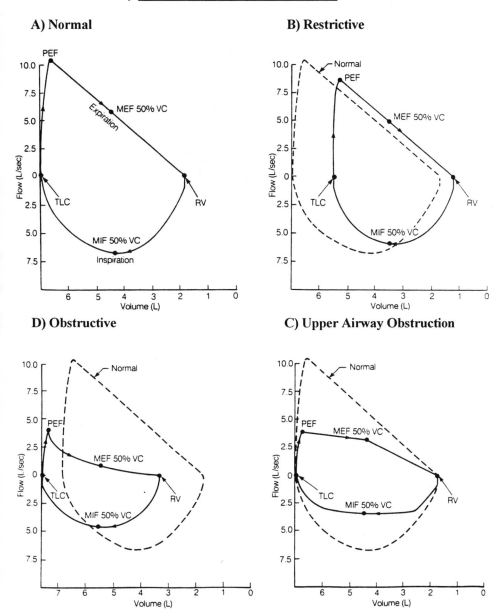

From *The Merck Manual of Diagnosis and Therapy*, 16th edition, pp. 611-612, edited by R. Berkow.

Copyright 1992 by Merck & Co., Inc., Rahway, NJ. Used with permission.

5.3.) <u>RESTRICTIVE LUNG DISEASES</u>

pneumoconiosis	- **silicosis** (quartz) - **anthracosis** (coal) - **asbestosis** (fibrous mineral) - **berylliosis** (metal)
drug induced pulm. fibrosis	- bleomycin - alkylating agents - oxygen therapy
hypersensitivity pneumonitis	- **farmer's lung** (actinomyces) - **cotton worker's lung** (byssinosis) - **pigeon breeder's lung** (animal protein) - **chemicals:** - isocyanide - vinyl chloride
Löffler's syndrome	- pulmonary infiltrate - unknown cause - eosinophilia

 Asbestos related diseases : - ***asbestosis***: *interstitial fibrosis*
                                    - ***mesothelioma***: *long latency, lethal*
                                    - ***bronchogenic carcinoma***: *5-100 x risk*

 "Honeycomb lung" = *late stage interstitial fibrosis (any cause).*

5.4.) <u>OBSTRUCTIVE LUNG DISEASES - 1</u>

emphysema	- loss of elastic recoil - imbalance of proteases and antiproteases - homozygotic deficiency of α1-antitrypsin
chronic bronchitis	- persistent, productive cough - at least 3 months each year - at least for 3 years
"classic" asthma	- episodic wheezing - intermittent cough - triggered by exposure to **specific allergens** - IgE mediated mast cell degranulation
intrinsic asthma	- generalized airway hypersensitivity - triggered by **non-allergenic factors**: irritants, infections, cold, exercise etc.

 Many patients have combined elements of chronic bronchitis, asthma and emphysema (chronic obstructive pulmonary disease).

5.5.) <u>OBSTRUCTIVE LUNG DISEASES - 2</u>

atelectasis	- following airway obstruction **acute**: pain, dyspnea, cyanosis blood pressure drop **chronic**: often asymptomatic
bronchiectasis	- chronic cough, foul sputum - hemoptysis - chronic bronchopulmonary infections - cystic fibrosis - immotile cilia syndrome (Kartagener's)
cystic fibrosis	**usual presentation**: - meconium plug, bowel obstruction - pancreatic insufficiency, steatorrhea - predisposition to infections, especially Pseudomonas - elevated sweat chloride - sterility in men - low fertility in women

5.6.) <u>PLEURAL EFFUSIONS</u>

exudate	transudate
protein > 3g/dl **pleural/serum protein > 0.5**	**protein < 3g/dl** **pleural/serum protein < 0.5**
- infections - malignancy - pulmonary embolism	- congestive heart failure - nephrotic syndrome - liver failure

5.7.) <u>SARCOIDOSIS & TUBERCULOSIS</u>

sarcoidosis	tuberculosis
- bilateral hilar lymphadenopathy - non-caseating granulomas **organ involvement:** - liver - spleen - eyes - skin (erythema nodosum)	**primary** - usually asymptomatic - hilar lymphadenopathy - Ghon complex : calcified peripheral nodule plus calcified hilar lymph node **secondary (reactivation)** - multiple foci in apical areas of lung - primary focus often undetectable **generalized (miliary)** - fever, weightloss, fatigue - hematogenous dissemination - pleurisy, pericarditis - meningitis - genitourinary involvement - bone and joint involvement - Pott's disease: tbc of spine

5.8.) PNEUMONIA: EPIDEMIOLOGY

A) COMMUNITY ACQUIRED

S. pneumoniae	- the "classic" one - still most common cause if community acquired - elderly, chronic illness, COPD, cigarettes
Hemophilus	- same epidemiology as S. pneumoniae
Legionella	- contaminated aerosols, air coolers etc.
Mycoplasma pneumoniae	- adolescents, young adults - colleges, boarding houses etc.

B) HOSPITAL ACQUIRED

gram negative bacilli	**- more than 50% of cases**
Pseudomonas aeruginosa	- faucets, sinks, ventilators, endoscopes
Staphylococcus aureus	- burn units, wound infections
Legionella	- water supply

C) UNUSUAL CAUSES

anthrax	- cattle, swine, horses
coccidoidomycosis	- San Joaquin valley (Southeast US)
hanta virus	- rodent droppings
histoplasmosis	- bat droppings, (river valleys of Southeast US)
leptospirosis	- water contaminated with animal urine
plague	- rats, squirrels (Western US)
psittacosis	- birds (parrots, pigeons...)
tularemia	- hunters (rabbits, foxes...)

5.9.) <u>PNEUMONIA: ENTITIES</u>

BACTERIAL	**bronchopneumonia** - patchy, peribronchial distribution - more common in infants and elderly **lobar pneumonia** - diffuse involvement of entire lobe - more common in middle age adults
- Pneumococci	- sudden onset fever, chills, dyspnea
- Klebsiella	- currant jelly sputum

- Legionella	- diffuse patchy infiltrate on chest x-ray
	- over 50 strains, wide spectrum of disease severity
	  ranging from acute, self-limited (Pontiac fever) to
	  high mortality form (Legionnaires' disease)

- Pseudomonas	- common in cystic fibrosis patients
ATYPICAL	**viral or mycoplasma** - interstitial pneumonia - spares intra-alveolar spaces
FUNGAL	**pneumocystis carinii** - only seen in immunocompromised patients - diffuse bilateral consolidation of lungs - often presents with persistent, dry cough - diagnosis: sputum (silver stain), biopsy

---

<u>*What is atypical about "atypical pneumonia"?*</u>
- *more gradual onset*
- *dry, non productive cough*
- *minimal signs of pulmonary involvement during physical examination*
- *prominent chest x-ray ("looks worse than patient")*
- *prominent extrapulmonary symptoms, myalgia etc.*

5.10.) <u>SLEEP APNEA</u>

central	obstructive
- sudden cessation of respiratory effort	- paradoxical motion of abdomen and rib cage during apneic episode - snoring - obesity, adenoids, macroglossia - Pickwickian syndrome

5.11.) <u>LUNG TUMORS</u>

squamous cell carcinoma (35%)	- **central location**
adenocarcinoma (35%)	- **peripheral location**
large cell carcinoma (15%)	- central or peripheral lesion - **tends to cavitate** - poor prognosis
small cell carcinoma (15%)	- usually central location - early involvement of mediastinum - **paraneoplastic syndromes** (in 10%) - poorest prognosis of all
carcinoid (5%)	- often **curable** by resection - usually endocrinologically silent - not a/w smoking

Stage I	- tumor 3 cm or less in diameter
Stage II	- tumor > 3 cm - or invades main bronchus - or invades visceral pleura
Stage III	- invades chest wall - or invades diaphragm
Stage IV	- invades mediastinum - or invades trachea or esophagus - or invades vertebral body - or shows pleural exudate

UPPER RESPIRATORY DISEASES

Common Cold
- no specific treatment
- nasal decongestants should not be used for more than a few days (may cause rhinitis medicamentosa)

Strep Throat
- antibiotics, mainly useful for preventing complications
- penicillin or erythromycin for 10 days
- if patient had rheumatic fever: prophylaxis for 5-10 years

Tonsillitis
- see "Strep throat"
- if recurrent: tonsillectomy
- if peritonsillar abscess develops: drain and parenteral antibiotics

Influenza
- bed rest, analgesics
- amantadine may shorten duration of symptoms
- if fever persists or WBC > 12000 suspect bacterial superinfection (antibiotics)

Sinusitis
- most commonly maxillary
- confirm with x-ray or coronal CT
- nasal decongestants, amoxicillin
- purulent discharge should be cultured
- failure to resolve: hospitalization, drainage

Epiglottitis
- hospitalization
- IV antibiotics and steroids
- intubation (always indicated in children !)

LOWER RESPIRATORY DISEASES

Asthma
- baseline spirometry
- home peak flow monitoring if moderate to severe
- mild attack: nebulized β-agonists
- moderate attack: nebulized β-agonists and corticosteroids
- severe attack: nebulized β-agonists and systemic corticosteroids
- respiratory acidosis: intubate and ventilate !

Bronchiolitis
- viral cause in children under 2 years of age
- treatment supportive
- in adults probably due to immune reaction (postinfectious, autoimmune)
- steroids may be useful

Pneumonia
- chest x-ray for initial evaluation
- sputum culture often not useful
- empirical therapy based on clinical setting
  (community acquired vs. nosocomial)
- high mortality if nosocomial: treat early, broad spectrum antibiotics
- pleural effusion with empyema: tube thoracostomy

Bronchiectasis
- sputum smear and culture
- empirical therapy (amoxicillin, trimethoprim/sulfamethoxazole)
- bronchoscopy / surgery if massive hemoptysis

Tuberculosis

- prophylaxis: isoniazid for 6 to 12 months
- treatment: isoniazid plus rifampin for 6 months plus ethambutol or streptomycin for first 2 months
- treatment in AIDS patient: start immediately with 4 or 5 drug regimen !

Acute Respiratory Distress Syndrome

- chest x-ray, arterial blood gases, pulmonary wedge pressure
- ventilation, oxygen, PEEP

Atelectasis

- identify cause of bronchial obstruction
- x-ray, CT for exact location
- bronchoscopy if tumor or foreign body is suspected

Pulmonary Embolism

- thrombolytic agents only for massive embolism with shock
- anticoagulation (first heparin, then warfarin 3-6 months) to prevent further embolization
- consider vena cava umbrella if anticoagulation is contraindicated

Solitary pulmonary nodule

- if likely benign (distinct margins, central calcification): watch it
- if likely malignant (patient > 35 years, no calcifications): needle aspiration or resection

Lung Cancer

- Non-small cell carcinoma: Surgery, however most patients present with unresectable disease (tumor involving trachea or main stem bronchi, malignant effusions, wide spread metastases)
- adjuvant chemotherapy is disappointing
- Small cell carcinoma: combination chemotherapy
- Palliative therapy (for bronchial obstruction, bone metastases, superior vena cava syndrome etc.): Radiation

COPD

- stop smoking !
- home oxygen therapy if $PaO_2 < 55$ mmHG (saturation <88%)
- lung transplantation is still experimental and has high mortality

Emphysema

- bronchodilators
- anticholinergics (ipratropium)

Chronic Bronchitis

- mobilize secretions (aerosols, chest percussion - avoid cough suppressants)

INTERSTITIAL LUNG DISEASE

Sarcoidosis

- rule out other granulomatous diseases (tbc, berylliosis etc.)
- consider biopsy to rule out lymphoma
- corticosteroids if systemic signs are present (constitutional symptoms, skin or CNS involvement etc.)

Asbestosis

- smoking multiplies risk
- mortality mainly due to bronchogenic carcinoma
- mesothelioma: radiation, chemotherapy, surgery usually unsuccessful

Silicosis

- increased risk for tuberculosis: get annual PPD test

GASTROINTESTINAL DISEASES

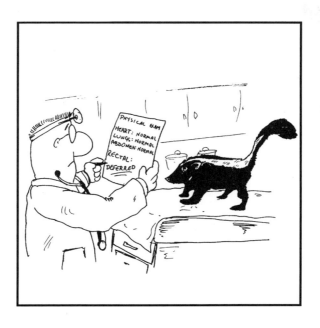

6.1.) GI FUNCTION TESTS

fecal fat	- quick test: Sudan III staining of stool smear - quantitative test: total fat in 3-day stool steatorrhea if > 6 g/day

xylose absorption test	- D-xylose is well absorbed but not metabolized
	- give oral D-xylose and measure amount
	   excreted in urine
	- low values indicate malabsorption
	   (e.g. bacterial overgrowth)

xylose breath test	- measure $^{14}CO_2$ in breath after ingestion of radioactive D-xylose - low values indicate malabsorption - more rapid to perform than the absorption test
bentiromide test	- administer synthetic peptide - measure arylamine in urine - indicates activity of pancreatic chymotrypsin
secretin test	- stimulate pancreas with secretin - measure volume and bicarbonate content of pancreatic secretion (duodenal aspirate)
Schilling test	measure radioactivity in 24h urine **Stage 1** after ingestion of radiolabeled vit. B12 **Stage 2** plus intrinsic factor **Stage 3** plus antibiotics

6.2.) GI BLEEDING

hematemesis	- vomiting bright, red blood **(rapid bleed)** - or "coffee-ground" like **(slow bleed)** - source: proximal to ligament of Treitz
melena	- black, tarry stool - source: **upper GI**, or lower GI to right colon
hematochezia	- bright red blood in stool - source: **lower GI**, or upper GI if massive

upper GI	lower GI	upper & lower GI
- esophageal varices - Mallory-Weiss - gastritis - gastric ulcer - duodenal ulcer	- hemorrhoids - anal fissure - diverticulosis - IBD - intussusception	- neoplasms - angiodysplasias (Osler's)

6.3.) <u>DYSPHAGIA</u>

achalasia	- dilated, fluid-filled esophagus - "bird beak" appearance on barium swallow - **high resting LES pressure** - *biopsy to exclude infiltrating gastric carcinoma !*
scleroderma (CREST)	- reflux, peptic strictures - **low resting LES pressure**
rings and webs	- congenital (Schatzki's rings) - or secondary to reflux disease - asymptomatic, or dysphagia for solids - **Plummer-Vinson:** webs + anemia + atrophic glossitis
carcinoma	**squamous cell carcinoma** <u>risk factors</u> - alcohol - tobacco - radiation - stasis (achalasia) **adenocarcinoma** - almost always from Barrett's esophagus

---

<u>Dysphagia for solid foods and liquids:</u>
- *esophageal spasm*
- *scleroderma*
- *achalasia*

<u>Dysphagia for solids worse than liquids:</u>
- *obstruction*
- *peptic strictures*
- *cancer*

6.4.) <u>UPPER ABDOMINAL PAIN</u>

reflux esophagitis	- burning substernal pain - **after meals, at night** - may radiate to left arm !
gastric ulcer	- steady, gnawing epigastric pain - **worsened by food**
duodenal ulcer	- steady, gnawing epigastric pain - typically awakens patient around 1:00 am - **relieved by food**
perforated peptic ulcer	- severe epigastric pain - may radiate to back or shoulders - emergency !
cholecystitis	- cramp-like epigastric pain - may radiate to tip of right scapula - Murphy's sign
acute pancreatitis	- severe, boring abdominal pain - often radiates to back - peritoneal signs

6.5.) <u>LOWER ABDOMINAL PAIN</u>

inflammatory bowel disease	- chronic, cramping pain - diarrhea, blood and pus in stool
intestinal obstruction	- hyperactive bowel sounds
intestinal infarction	- absent bowel sounds - gross or occult blood in stool
appendicitis	- vague periumbilical pain, nausea - later localizes to lower right quadrant - perforation: high fever and leukocytosis
diverticulitis	- steady pain - localized to lower left quadrant -"left sided appendicitis"

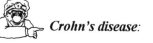

Crohn's disease: - *chronic cramping pain*
                     - *fever, anorexia, weight loss*

Ulcerative colitis: - *less abdominal pain*
                        - *more bloody diarrhea*

98

6.6.) <u>STOMACH & DUODENUM</u>

acute gastritis (erosive)	- acute hemorrhagic lesions - stress ulcers - aspirin, NSAIDs - alcohol
chronic gastritis A (non-erosive)	- **autoimmune gastritis** - body and fundus - pernicious anemia
chronic gastritis B (non-erosive)	- **infectious gastritis** - body and antrum - H. pylori
gastric ulcer	- **normal or decreased acid** production - decreased mucosal resistance - NSAIDs
duodenal ulcer	- **increased acid** production - H. pylori

6.7.) <u>MALDIGESTION</u>

maldigestion	malabsorption
dysfunction of exocrine pancreas - chronic pancreatitis - cystic fibrosis **deficiency of specific enzymes** - lactase deficiency **lack of bile salts** - biliary cirrhosis - resected terminal ileum - bacterial overgrowth	**dysfunction of small bowel** - short bowel syndrome - bacterial overgrowth - celiac disease - tropical sprue - Whipple's disease **dysfunction of specific transporters** - cystinuria - Hartnup disease

	Diagnostic Clues
celiac disease	- iron deficiency anemia that doesn't respond to oral iron - **jejunal biopsy**: flat mucosa
tropical sprue	- diarrhea and megaloblastic anemia several months after travel to tropical country - **jejunal biopsy**: broad and flat villi, inflammation
Whipple's disease	- polyarthritis - abnormal skin pigmentation, - lymphadenopathy - **jejunal biopsy**: PAS positive granules in macrophages

6.8.) PANCREATITIS

acute pancreatitis	chronic pancreatitis
a/w **alcohol abuse** a/w **cholelithiasis** complication of ERCP	a/w **alcohol abuse** rarely a/w cholelithias
- **elevated serum amylase** - if normal needs to be confirmed by CT	- **serum amylase often normal** - pancreatic calcifications

10% mortality rate	- endocrine insufficiency
	  (NIDDM)
	- exocrine insufficiency
	  (maldigestion)

> *Complications of pancreatitis:*
> - *fat necrosis*
> - *respiratory distress syndrome*
> - *acute tubular necrosis*
> - *hemorrhage, DIC*
> - *pancreatic abscess*
> - *pancreatic pseudocysts*
> - *pancreas insufficiency*

> *Signs of poor prognosis:*
> - *white blood cells > 16,000 / mm^3*
> - *fall in hematocrit by > 10%*
> - *serum calcium < 8 mg/dl*

6.9.) <u>SIGNS OF LIVER DISEASE</u>

jaundice	- diminished bilirubin secretion
fetor hepaticus	- sulfur compounds produced by intestinal bacteria, not cleared by liver
spider angiomas **palmar erythema** **gynecomastia**	- elevated estrogen levels
ecchymoses	- decreased synthesis of clotting factors
xanthomas	- elevated cholesterol levels
hypoglycemia	- decreased glycogen stores - decreased neoglucogenesis
hypersplenism	- portal hypertension
encephalopathy **asterixis**	- portosystemic shunt
hepatorenal syndrome **(decline of GFR)**	- renal failure of unknown pathogenesis - kidneys are normal ! (may be transplanted) - a/w severe ascites - usually fatal

- liver cell damage:	*AST, ALT*
- bile duct obstruction:	*alkaline phosphatase*
- cholestasis:	*γ-GT*

6.10.) <u>HEPATITIS A</u>

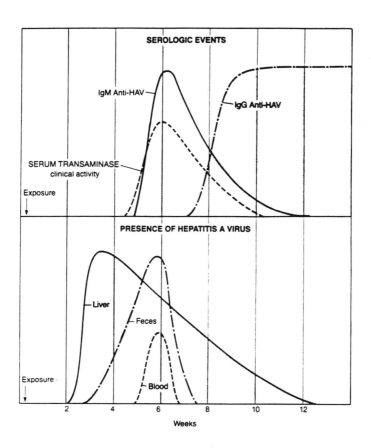

From *Pathology*, 2nd edition, p. 722, edited by E. Rubin and J.L. Farber.
Copyright 1994 by J.B. Lippincott Co., Philadelphia, PA. Used with permission.

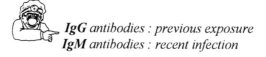

IgG antibodies : previous exposure
IgM antibodies : recent infection

6.11.) HEPATITIS B

HBsAg	- "Australia antigen" - indicates **acute or chronic infection** - used for blood bank screening
HBeAg	- indicates high degree of **infectivity**
anti-HBc	- **earliest indicator of acute infection** [1]
anti-HBe	- indicates **resolution** of acute infection
anti-HBs	- indicates **immunity** (post-infection or post vaccination)

[1] HBsAg and HBeAg appear earlier but are more difficult and expensive to determine

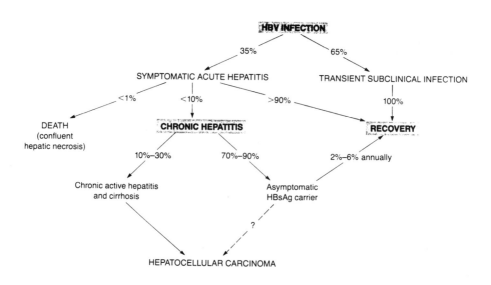

From *Pathology*, 2nd edition, p. 726, edited by E. Rubin and J.L. Farber.
Copyright 1994 by J.B. Lippincott Co., Philadelphia, PA. Used with permission.

6.12.) <u>MORE HEPATITIS B</u>

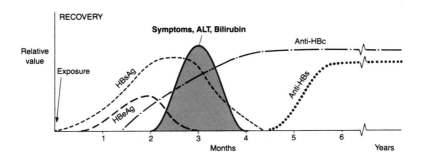

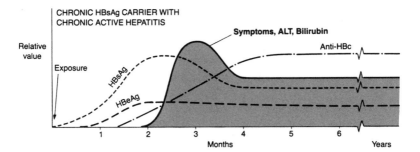

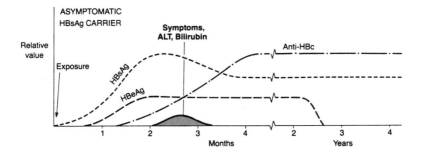

From *Pathology*, 2nd edition, p. 725, edited by E. Rubin and J.L. Farber.
Copyright 1994 by J.B. Lippincott Co., Philadelphia, PA. Used with permission.

6.13.) <u>DRUG INDUCED LIVER DISEASE</u>

estrogens **chlorpromazine**	- reversible cholestasis
ethanol	- fatty liver - cirrhosis (initially micro-, later macronodular)
acetaminophen **carbon tetrachloride**	- liver cell necrosis
estrogens	- hepatocellular adenoma (benign)
aflatoxin **hepatitis B and C**	- hepatocellular carcinoma
vinyl chloride **arsenic**	- angiosarcoma

 Chronic liver failure increases systemic
concentration of many drugs due to:
- *decreased P450 function*
- *decreased first-pass effect (porto-caval shunt)*
- *hypoalbuminemia*

6.14.) GALLBLADDER

gallstones	**- 75% cholesterol stones** **- 25% pigment stones** maybe asymptomatic (70%) may cause biliary colic (20%) may cause cholecystitis (10%)
biliary colic	- steady, cramplike (non-colicky !) pain in epigastrium - pain <u>subsides over 30-60 min.</u>
cholecystitis	- steady, cramplike pain in epigastrium - **Murphy's sign** (inspiratory arrest during palpation) - pain <u>does not subside spontaneously</u>

cholangitis	**Charcot's triad** : - biliary pain
	                  - jaundice
	                  - fever

sclerosing cholangitis	- autoimmune inflammation of the bile ducts - rare complication of ulcerative colitis

6.15.) DIARRHEA: TYPES

secretory	**- large volume watery stools** **- persists with fasting** - cholera - carcinoid - VIP secreting tumors
osmotic	**- bulky, greasy stools** **- improves with fasting** - lactase deficiency - pancreatic insufficiency - short bowel syndrome
inflammatory	**- frequent but small stools** **- blood and/or pus** - inflammatory bowel disease - irradiation - shigella, amebiasis
dysmotility	**- diarrhea alternating with constipation** - irritable bowel syndrome - diabetes mellitus

 Diarrhea of any cause may lead to transient lactase deficiency.

6.16.) <u>DIARRHEA: DIAGNOSTIC CLUES</u>

right lower quadrant mass	- Crohn's
arthritis	- ulcerative colitis - Crohn's - Whipple's
significant weight loss	- cancer - malabsorption - IBD
purpura	- celiac disease
eosinophilia	- parasitic disease
flushing	- carcinoid
lymphadenopathy immunosuppression	- AIDS (Gardiasis)

 Bismuth subsalicylate may prevent infection with enterotoxin producing E. coli. Great for travelers to exotic countries like Indonesia.

6.17.) <u>INFLAMMATORY BOWEL DISEASE</u>

Crohn's disease	ulcerative colitis
skip lesions (segmental inflammation) transmural	continuous inflammatory process mucosa / submucosa only
granulomas strictures and fissures	crypt abscesses pseudopolyps
rectum often spared ileum often involved	begins at rectum and progresses towards ileocecal junction
cramping abdominal pain	**frequent bloody stools**
	increased risk for colon carcinoma

<u>*Common extraintestinal manifestations*</u>*:*
- *arthritis*
- *sacroilitis*
- *sclerosing cholangitis*
- *iritis, conjunctivitis*
- *erythema nodosum*

6.18.) <u>COLORECTAL CANCER</u>

		5 year survival
Duke A	- limited to mucosa	95 %
Duke B	- extends to serosa	65 %
Duke C	- extends to regional lymph nodes	30 %
Duke D	- distant metastases	5%

DIGESTIVE DISEASES

Diarrhea
- symptomatic treatment (opiate) except in IBD and acute infections
- if chronic or patient very ill (fever, bloody diarrhea): get stool exam for white blood cells, ova, parasites, stool culture, *Clostridium difficile* toxin and liver function tests.
- Next consider endoscopy

Constipation
- eat fiber, discourage laxatives (except bulk-forming agents)
- exclude metabolic disorders: hypokalemia, diabetes mellitus, hypothyroidism
- drug history (anticholinergic side effects !)

Obesity
- body mass index: weight / height^2 (normal 20-25 kg/m^2)
- behavior modification
- exercise
- yo-yo dieting may be a/w increased risk for coronary artery disease
- surgery (gastroplasty, gastric bypass) only for severe obesity (BMI > 40)

Anorexia Nervosa
- hospitalization
- psychotherapy
- restore normal eating pattern
- force feeding only in life threatening situation
- mortality about 5%

Kwashiorkor/Marasmus
- watch for electrolyte imbalances
- don't refeed too rapidly !

ESOPHAGUS

Dysphagia
- barium swallow distinguishes between obstructive and motility disorders
- manometry if obstructions have been excluded
- endoscopy is study of choice to evaluate persistent heartburn and obstructions

Achalasia
- nifedipine
- pneumatic dilation
- surgical myotomy if pneumatic dilation fails (caveat reflux !)

Reflux Esophagitis
- avoid irritant food (coffee, alcohol, peppermint, fried food)
- don't eat prior to bed time, elevate head of bed
- antacids for occasional "heartburn"
- H_2 antagonists for long term
- proton pump inhibitors only for short term therapy

Esophageal bleeding
- acute: balloon tube tamponade (Sengstaken)
- to prevent rebleeding: endoscopic sclerotherapy
- β-blockers reduce risk of bleeding
- portosystemic shunts have lower rebleeding rate than sclerotherapy but significant incidence of encephalopathy

Esophageal Cancer
- if detected early (very rare): en-block resection
- palliative: radiation, chemotherapy, endoscopically guided laser therapy

STOMACH

Acute Gastritis
- discontinue NSAIDs, or add misoprostol
- if bleeding caused by aspirin: consider platelet administration
- sucralfate / H_2 antagonists

Chronic Gastritis
- type A: treat pernicious anemia: monthly, lifelong IM injections of vit. B12
- type B: eradicate H. pylori: combination of 2 or 3 antibiotics

Peptic Ulcer Disease
- eradicate H. pylori: antibiotics plus proton pump inhibitor
- endoscopic biopsy to exclude adenocarcinoma of the stomach
- if refractory: obtain fasting serum gastrin levels to exclude Zollinger-Ellison.
- Consider parietal cell vagotomy. Partial gastrectomy with gastro-duodenostomy (Billroth-I) or gastrojejunostomy (Billroth-II) are rarely used nowadays.

Stomach Cancer
- adenocarcinoma: resect if possible
- lymphoma: resect if limited to stomach, otherwise chemotherapy

INTESTINE

Appendicitis
- CBC with white cell differential
- determine hCG to exclude pregnancy if female
- peritoneal signs indicate surgical intervention

Diverticulitis
- don't perform barium enema during acute attack !
- liquid diet, antibiotics
- consider nasogastric suction and IV antibiotics if severe
- resection if perforated

Peritonitis
- abdominal film: air under diaphragm indicates perforation
- IV antibiotics
- surgery to drain abscess or repair perforation etc.

Malabsorption
- celiac sprue: gluten free diet (rice and corn are o.k.)
- rule out lymphoma (late complication)
- tropical sprue (usually Klebsiella or E. coli): antibiotics
- Whipple's disease (Tropheryma whippelii): tetracycline

Ulcerative Colitis
- sulfasalazine (5-ASA bound to sulfapyridine) for mild to moderate UC
- sulfasalazine reduces relapse rate
- topical or systemic steroids for acute attacks
- opiates and anticholinergics are contraindicated
- surgical treatment is curative

Crohn's Disease
- sulfasalazine (note: newer 5-ASA preparations have fewer side effects)
- sulfasalazine does not reduce relapse rate
- systemic steroids for acute attacks
- 6-mercaptopurine (azathioprine) may allow reduction of steroid dose
- avoid surgery if possible. Most patients who have been operated will require more and more additional surgery

Toxic Megacolon
- nasogastric suction
- broad spectrum antibiotics cover
- if it worsens: surgery to prevent perforation

Irritable Bowel Syndrome
- rule out lactase deficiency
- try high fiber diet
- anticholinergics and antidiarrhea drugs are useful
- anxiolytics and narcotics should be avoided because of their addictive potential

Colon Polyps
- if polyp is found by sigmoidoscopy and biopsy shows hyperplastic polyp (benign), no further workup is needed
- if biopsy shows adenomatous polyp: perform colonoscopy to identify and remove additional polyps
- if colonoscopy shows polyposis: screen all family members

Colon Cancer
- surgical resection
- adjuvant chemotherapy for Duke C and D
- follow-up: monitor CEA

LIVER

Viral Hepatitis
- bed rest as needed
- consider IV glucose if severe nausea and vomiting present
- steroids of little or no benefit
- chronic hepatitis: recombinant human interferon α
- infectious patient: isolate if patient with hepatitis A or E has fecal incontinence or patient with hepatitis B is bleeding
- asymptomatic carriers: Perinatal transmission ! Sexual transmission !

Cirrhosis

- alcohol abstinence
- reduce dietary protein if encephalopathy develops
- ascites: reduce by 2-3 lbs/day (salt restriction, diuretics). Large volume paracentesis (4-5 lbs/day) requires albumin supplementation to protect intravascular volume
- vit. K to correct bleeding tendency may be ineffective in severe liver failure
- liver transplantation in suitable patients

Liver Cancer

- hepatocellular carcinoma: resect solitary nodule. Chemotherapy of little benefit
- liver cell adenoma: May regress following cessation of oral contraceptives. Otherwise resect if possible

Cholelithiasis

- no need for surgery in asymptomatic patient (except porcelain gallbladder)
- if symptomatic: laparoscopic cholecystectomy
- bile salts (ursodeoxycholic acid etc.) for small <u>cholesterol</u> stones

Cholecystitis

- withhold oral food
- antibiotics
- analgesics (avoid morphine -> spasm of Oddi's sphincter)
- if symptoms don't subside within a few days: definite surgery

PANCREAS

Acute Pancreatitis

- no food or liquids by mouth
- nasogastric suction
- ERCP and endoscopic sphincterotomy if due to choledocholithiasis
- surgery if pancreatic necrosis develops

Chronic Pancreatitis
- stop alcohol
- low fat diet
- dietary enzyme supplement (lipase, amylase, protease)
- surgical correction of cholelithiasis, choledocholithiasis, stenosis of sphincter of Oddi

EMERGENCIES

Acute Abdomen
- parenteral analgesics or narcotics
- antibiotics only if definite signs of systemic infection are present
- **emergency surgery indicated for**: perforation (peptic ulcer, bowel), intestinal strangulation, suppurative cholangitis, ruptured aortic aneurysm, mesenteric thrombosis, rupture of spleen, rupture of ectopic pregnancy
- **surgery may be delayed or is unnecessary for**: biliary colic, acute cholecystitis, splenic infarct, renal infarct, acute pancreatitis, ruptured ovarian follicle cyst

Paralytic Ileus
- restrict oral intake
- nasogastric suction if prolonged

Upper GI Bleeding
- evaluate hemodynamic status, stabilize
- nasogastric tube
- endoscopy if bleeding is severe enough to require blood transfusions
- bleeding from esophageal varices: endoscopic sclerotherapy preferred

Lower GI Bleeding
- evaluate hemodynamic status, stabilize
- colonoscopy if bleeding is severe or patient > 50 years (neoplasms)
- if bleeding continues consider ^{99m}TC red cell scan or mesenteric angiography (often limited if bleeding slow or intermittent)

UROGENITAL DISEASES

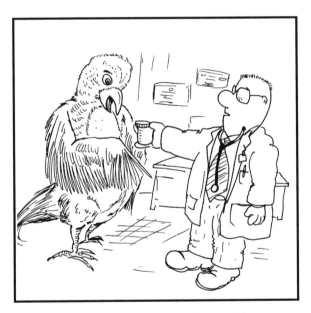

"What's a urine specimen?"

7.1.) URINE

pH	- **acidic**: high protein diet
	              ketoacidosis (diabetes, starvation)
	- **alkaline**: urinary tract infections
	             renal tubular acidosis

reducing substances	- **glucose, fructose, galactose** - false positive: Vit. C, salicylates
ketones	- dip sticks detect **acetone** and **acetoacetic** acid but not β-hydroxybutyric acid

casts	- **RBC** : acute glomerulonephritis
	           malignant hypertension
	
	- **WBC** : pyelonephritis
	
	- **hyaline** : a few are normal
	             low urinary flow
	             hypertension
	
	- **fatty** : nephrotic syndrome
	- **granular** : acute tubular necrosis
	- **waxy** : advanced chronic renal disease

creatinine clearance	- most sensitive indicator of renal function (GFR)
	  (needs to be adjusted for body size in children)
	
	- to monitor patients who take nephrotoxic drugs
	- to determine dosage of drugs when serum level
	  depends critically on renal clearance

7.2.) UROLITHIASIS

calcium	- 75% of cases - precipitates in <u>alkaline</u> urine - **opaque, round, multiple** - hypercalciuria - hyperoxaluria
Mg - NH$_3$ - Phosphate	- 20% of cases - "triple stones" - precipitates in <u>alkaline</u> urine - **opaque, form staghorn calculi** - following infection by urease positive bacteria (e.g. Proteus)
uric acid	- 5% of cases - precipitates in **acidic** urine - **radiolucent stones** - gout - leukemia

cystine	- precipitates in **acidic** urine
	
	- **opaque, form staghorn calculi**
	- hypercystinuria
	  (congenital defect in dibasic
	    amino acid transporter)

7.3.) <u>AZOTEMIA</u>

	prerenal	renal
urine osmolality	> 500	< 250
urine Na$^+$	< 10	> 20
fractional excreted Na$^+$	< 1	> 1
casts	hyaline	brown, granular

- azotemia = nitrogen retention (BUN > 20 mg/dl , creatinine > 1.5 mg/dl)

- may present with oliguria (<400 ml/24h) or normal urine output

 fractional excretion of Na$^+$ is calculated relative to creatinine:

$$FE_{Na} = (U_{Na} / P_{Na}) / (U_{cr} / P_{cr})$$

7.4.) <u>ACUTE RENAL FAILURE</u>

prerenal	**low cardiac output**
	hypovolemia - hemorrhage - burns - sequestration
	systemic vasodilation - sepsis - anaphylaxis

renal	**acute tubular necrosis**
	- ischemia
	- toxins: aminoglycosides
	            iodinated contrast agents,
	            cadmium
	            cisplatin

	acute interstitial nephritis - drugs: β-lactams sulfonamides
	acute glomerulonephritis **acute pyelonephritis** **rhabdomyolysis** (crash injury)
postrenal	**obstruction** - ureter calculi, tumors - urethra strictures - neurogenic bladder

 ARF : *oliguria (<400 ml/d)*
azotemia

ATN : *most but not all cases of ARF due to ATN*
characteristic dirty brown granular casts

7.5.) <u>CHRONIC RENAL FAILURE</u>

uremia [1]	- increased BUN, increased creatinine - urine volume may be low or normal - anemia (normocytic, normochromic) - bleeding tendency - peripheral neuropathy - encephalopathy
hypertriglyceridemia	- increased production of triglycerides - cholesterol levels normal - premature atherosclerosis
metabolic acidosis	- urinary pH often normal - reduction in NH_3 synthesis (nontitratable acid) limits H^+ excretion - **anion gap** due to retention of phosphates etc.

osteodystrophy
(secondary hyperparathyroidism)
	- **decreased excretion of phosphate**
	  (-> hyperphosphatemia, binds calcium)
	- **decreased synthesis of 1.25$(OH)_2$D**
	  (->decreased intestinal absorption of calcium)
	  -> hypocalcemia -> increases PTH
	
	usually more severe in children:
	- subperiosteal erosions, bone cysts
	  (especially phalanges)
	- widened osteoid seams (renal rickets)

[1] the term "uremia" in clinical usage refers to the signs and symptoms of chronic renal failure. Azotemia (increased levels of nitrogenous compounds) is an <u>early</u> sign of uremia.

most common causes of chronic kidney failure:
- *hypertension*
- *diabetes*
- *glomerulonephritis*

7.6.) <u>DRUG USAGE IN RENAL FAILURE</u>

(partial list of most common medications)

avoid	reduce dosage
- IV contrast studies - sulfonylureas - tetracyclines (except doxycycline)	- digoxin - quinidine - aminoglycosides - cimetidine - lithium

7.7.) <u>DRUG INDUCED NEPHROPATHY</u>

penicillin **sulfonamides** **rifampin**	- acute interstitial nephritis
NSAIDs (especially phenacetin)	- chronic interstitial nephritis with nephrotic syndrome
cyclosporin A	- renal vasospasm

125

7.8.) <u>NEPHRITIC & NEPHROTIC</u>

nephritic syndrome	nephrotic syndrome
- RBC casts - hematuria	- proteinuria - hypoalbuminemia - hyperlipidemia - edema

acute nephritic: - poststreptococcal
- Goodpasture
- SLE
- Henoch-Schönlein

nephritic/nephrotic: - membranoproliferative
- SLE
- Henoch-Schönlein

nephrotic: - minimal change (children)
- membraneous (adults)

7.9.) GLOMERULAR DISEASE - 1

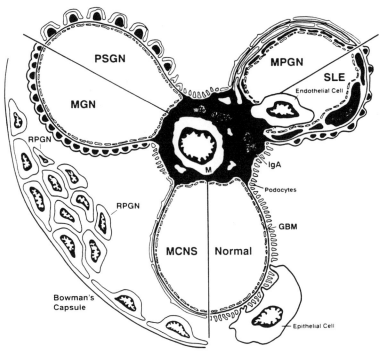

From *Cecil Essentials of Medicine*, 3rd edition, p. 213, edited by T.E. Andreoli et al.
Copyright 1993 by W.B. Saunders Co., Philadelphia, PA. Used with permission.

PSGN: Post-streptococcal   **MPGN**: Membrano-proliferative   **MGN**: Membranous
RPGN: Rapidly progressive   **MCNS**: Minimal change   **SLE**: Lupus erythematosus
IgA: IgA deposits in IgA nephropathy

M: Mesangium   **GBM**: glomerular basement membrane

Goodpasture's (anti-GBM antibodies)	- young males - pulmonary hemorrhage
Berger's (IgA nephropathy)	- same as Henoch Schönlein - may follow resp. infection - hematuria - mild proteinuria, hematuria

7.10.) GLOMERULAR DISEASE - 2

			prognosis
minimal change (lipoid nephrosis)	- most common nephrotic syndrome in children - insidious onset	- no immune complexes - **loss of foot processes in EM.**	good
membranous	- most common nephrotic syndrome in young adults - insidious onset	- LM. : thickening of GBM - **subepithelial deposits of** immune complexes - 85% unknown antigen	mixed
membrano proliferative	- variable presentation	- GBM thickening plus proliferation of mesangium - **subendothelial or intra-membranous** deposits of immune complexes - "tram track" appearance	very poor
focal segmental	- maybe related to minimal change - but proteinuria is nonselective	- segmental sclerosis - usually IgM deposits **(IgA in Berger's)**	poor
diffuse proliferative	- nephritic/nephrotic - **post streptococcal, SLE**	- proliferation of mesangium and epithelium - **subepithelial deposits**	good
rapidly progressive	- aggressive variant of other GN	- **crescents** - oliguria, uremia	very poor

7.11.) <u>SCROTUM & TESTES</u>

hydrocele	- painless - **transilluminates** - sometimes a/w testicular tumors !
varicocele	- contorted, dilated veins - feels like a "**bag of worms**" - may cause infertility - empties with patient in supine position
torsion of testes	- acute pain and swelling - affected **testis typically lies higher** - primarily affects teenagers
epididymo-orchitis	- acute pain, nausea, fever - **pain relief upon elevation of scrotum**
testicular cancer	- usually painless mass - sometimes may resemble epididymitis - **spreads very easily (avoid vigorous palpation or biopsy !)**

7.12.) <u>PROSTATE CANCER</u>

Stage A	- incidental finding (autopsy or biopsy) - non-palpable
Stage B	- palpable tumor - does not extend beyond capsule
Stage C	- extends beyond capsule - no evidence of metastases
Stage D	- pelvic lymph nodes - metastases

- *prostate carcinoma is the most common carcinoma in the male.*
- *localized (curable) carcinoma in 60% of cases.*
- *metastasizes to bones (back pain may be the first symptom of advanced disease !)*

Hot-List

KIDNEYS

Stones
- morphine or meperidine for colic
- surgical removal or lithotripsy of obstructing stones
- uric acid stones can be resolved by urine alkalinization, all others cannot be chemically resolved
- screen for electrolyte abnormalities (Ca, phosphate, citrate, oxalate, uric acid)
- double daily fluid intake to prevent recurrence

Acute Renal Failure
- determine urinary indices to distinguish prerenal, renal and postrenal disease
- absence of hydronephrosis on renal ultrasound excludes obstruction
- **prerenal azotemia**: restore kidney perfusion
- **acute tubular necrosis**: convert oliguric to nonoliguric state (mannitol, loop diuretics). Restrict fluid, electrolytes and protein. Consider dialysis

Chronic Renal Failure
- Restrict salt and water, restrict potassium, phosphate and magnesium
- start dialysis if creatinine > 10 mg/dl or BUN > 100 mg/dl
- most patients prefer peritoneal dialysis over hemodialysis

Pyelonephritis
- obtain urine and blood cultures
- empirical IV ampicillin plus aminoglycoside

Acute Nephritic Syndrome
- ASO titer
- no specific therapy for poststreptococcal GN (steroids don't help)
- salt restriction or diuretics only if edema present

Nephrotic Syndrome
- <u>reduce</u> protein intake, unless negative protein balance results in malnutrition
- salt restriction. Loop diuretic if patient remains edematous
- watch for hypercoagulability due to loss of antithrombin III (may require heparin)
- specific treatment (responsiveness to steroids) depends on renal biopsy

Rapidly Progressive GN
- early biopsy is essential
- steroids and cytotoxic drugs
- plasmapheresis to remove anti-basement antibodies

BLADDER

Cystitis
- trimethoprim-sulfamethoxazole
- quinolones

Cancer
- transurethral resection or intravesical chemotherapy if carcinoma in situ or early stage (5%)
- chemotherapy if late stage or lymph nodes involved (95%)

MALE REPRODUCTIVE ORGANS

Erectile Impotence
- exclude neurological disease, vascular disease, diabetes mellitus
- nocturnal tumescence study !!!
- oral yohimbine works (somewhat)
- vacuum suction device
- penile prosthesis

Urethritis

- check for other STDs (blood serology for syphilis etc.)
- ceftriaxone for gonorrheal urethritis
- plus tetracycline for non-gonorrheal urethritis (often coexisting chlamydia)

Epididymitis

- bed rest, scrotal support
- systemic antibiotics

Hydrocele

- aspiration may cause secondary infertility
- surgical excision if large and symptomatic

Varicocele

- surgical excision if large and symptomatic (improves fertility)

Torsion of Testis

- immediate surgery, preventive fixation of <u>both</u> testes

Testicular Cancer

- seminoma (local): orchiectomy plus radiation
- seminoma with positive lymph nodes: orchiectomy plus chemotherapy
- non-seminoma: orchiectomy plus lymph node dissection plus chemotherapy

Benign Prostate Hyperplasia

- determine postvoid residual urine and PSA
- terazosin (α_1 - blocker)
- finasteride (blocks conversion of testosterone to DHT)
- transurethral resection

Prostate Carcinoma

- if <u>localized</u>:
  radical prostatectomy or radiation therapy or observation
- for <u>metastatic disease</u>
  androgen deprivation: orchiectomy or antiandrogens or LHRH agonists,
  radiate bone metastases
  pain management

SEXUALLY TRANSMITTED DISEASES

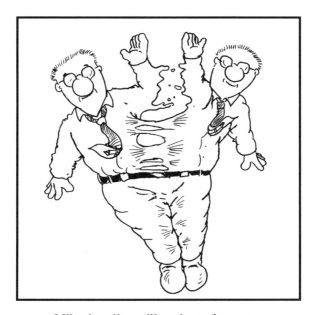

Mitosis – the ultimate safe sex.

8.1.) AIDS

1.) Definition (CDC revised 1993)

- HIV positive on ELISA and confirmed by Western blot
- plus   - CD4 < 200 cells/mm^3
          - or CD4 < 14%
          - or opportunistic disease

2.) Acute retroviral syndrome :   - fever
                                       - lymphadenopathy
                                       - malaise
                                       - sore throat
                                       - headache
                                       - nausea
                                       - weight loss

```
CD4 count : - check every 6 months if CD4 > 300
            - check every 3 months if CD4 < 300
            - start PCP prophylaxis if CD4 < 200
```

3.) AZT : - decreases rate of maternal/fetal transmission
             - delays progression of HIV infection
             - improves survival

      - side effects: - nausea, malaise
                         - muscle weakness
                         - anemia

```
- should be offered to symptomatic patients
- should be offered to asymptomatic patients if CD4 < 500
- could be considered for HIV positive patients with CD4 > 500
```

136

8.2.) <u>AIDS : MOST COMMON SYMPTOMS</u>

fever	- opportunistic **infections** - opportunistic **malignancies**
skin	- Herpes zoster - Candida - Kaposi sarcoma (homosexuals !)
cough	- **bacterial pneumonia** : lobar infiltrate - **P. carinii** : bilateral interstitial infiltrates or normal chest x-ray - **tuberculosis** : focal infiltrates, cavitary lesions or miliary
dyspnea	- exertional dyspnea plus dry cough: think Pneumocystis carinii !
dysphagia	- Candida - Herpes simplex - aphthous ulcers
diarrhea	- parasitic - bacterial (Campylobacter, Salmonella, Shigella)
headache	- bacterial meningitis - neurosyphilis - cryptococcosis - toxoplasmosis ("ring enhancing lesions") - if focal signs or altered mental status -> CT (contrast) or MRI - if scan normal : CSF for cryptococcus and acid fast bacteria

 Earliest Symptoms :   *- generalized lymphadenopathy*
- oral lesions (thrush, leukoplakia)
- reactivation herpes zoster

8.3.) <u>AIDS : OPPORTUNISTIC INFECTIONS</u>
<u>(Prophylaxis)</u>

Pneumocystis carinii	- all patients with CD < 200 cells/mm^3 - prevention of recurrence - *trimethoprim-sulfamethoxazole* - *or dapsone* - *or pentamidine*
tuberculosis	- PPD (Mantoux): positive if > 5mm - anergy control (candida, mumps, tetanus) - *isoniazid for at least 1 year* - *or rifampin for at least 1 year*
Mycobacterium avium	- patients with CD < 200 cells/mm^3 - *rifabutin (development of resistance likely)*
toxoplasmosis	- patients with CD < 200 cells/mm^3 - *trimethoprim-sulfamethoxazole* - *or pyrimethamine*
neurosyphilis	- check VDRL titer once a year - if positive consider lumbar puncture to confirm - *aggressive treatment with penicillin G*

8.4.) <u>AIDS : OPPORTUNISTIC INFECTIONS</u>
<u>(Treatment)</u>

HSV	*acyclovir*
CMV	*ganciclovir*
Mycobacterium tuberculosis	*four drug regimen:* *- isoniazid* *- rifampin* *- pyrazinamide* *- ethambutol*
Candida	*clotrimazole*
Cryptococcus neoformans	*amphotericin B*
Pneumocystis carinii	*trimethoprim-sulfamethoxazole* *(pentamidine if allergic)*
Toxoplasma gondii	*pyrimethamine-sulfadiazine*

8.5.) OTHER SEXUALLY TRANSMITTED DISEASES

condyloma acuminatum	HPV	"red warts"	*cryotherapy*
syphilis (I) **syphilis (II)** **syphilis (III)**	Treponema pallidum	hard chancre **(painless)** cond. lata (flat brown papules) gumma	*penicillin G*
chancroid	Hemophilus ducreii	soft chancre **(painful)**	*ceftriaxone*
lymphogranuloma venerum	Chlamydia trachomatis	ulcer **(painless)** lymphadenopathy	*doxycycline*
granuloma inguinale	C. donovani	multiple ulcerating papules lymph nodes not involved [1]	*tetracycline*
trichomoniasis	Trichomonas vaginalis	men : asymptomatic or NGU female : vaginitis	*metronidazole*
genital herpes	HSV2 or HSV1	recurrent vesicles **(painful)**	*acyclovir*
candidiasis [2]	Candida albicans	female : vaginitis	*nystatin, niconazole*

[1] induration of subcutaneous tissue.   [2] listed here for comparison, but candidiasis is not considered to be a VD.

INFECTIOUS DISEASES

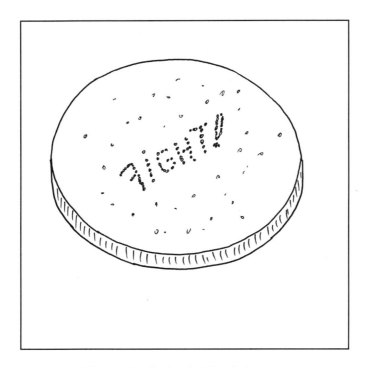

Bacterial Colonial Resistance

9.1.) <u>Key-List</u>

9.2.) <u>DEFENSE MECHANISMS</u>

skin barrier	- staphylococci - streptococci
IgA antibodies	- mucos membrane colonizing flora

cell-mediated immunity	**- bacteria**
	  M. tuberculosis
	  atypical mycobacteria
	- viruses
	- fungi
	- protozoae

neutrophils	- Staphylococci - Candida - Aspergillus

complement	**- encapsulated bacteria**
	  Streptococcus pneumoniae
	  Neisseria meningitis
	  Hemophilus influenzae

<u>*defective neutrophil function*</u>:
chronic granulomatous disease - NBT test, absent superoxide production
Chédiak-Higashi - reduced chemotaxis
Myeloperoxidase deficiency - enzyme defect

9.3.) <u>NOSOCOMIAL INFECTIONS</u>

urinary tract infections	- duration of catheterization - absence of systemic antibiotics - more common in females
lower respiratory tract infections	- aspiration - decreased gag reflex - alkaline stomach pH
surgical wound infections	- duration of procedure - level of contamination - severity of illness **recommended antibiotic prophylaxis**: 2 h before until 24 h after operation
sepsis *mortality about 25%*	**primary** - intravenous cannulas **secondary** - urinary tract infections - pulmonary infections - cutaneous infections - wound infections

9.4.) <u>FEVER PLUS RASH</u>

Rocky Mountain spotted fever	- maculopapular petechiae - beginning at wrist and forearm - spreading to trunk, palms, soles - **endemic areas :** Atlantic States, Southeast

Lyme disease	- erythema migrans
	  (expanding, annular erythema)
	- **endemic areas :**
	  Northeast, Minnesota, California, Oregon

meningococcal sepsis	- small petechia - irregular borders, "smudging" - painful - **outbreaks in military recruits (crowding)**
staphylococcal sepsis	- pustules, purulent purpura - nosocomial: indwelling catheters
pseudomonas sepsis	- hemorrhagic vesicles - patient extremely toxic
candida sepsis	- discrete, pink, maculopapular lesions - a/w **immunosuppresion** - a/w **broadspectrum antibiotics**
infective endocarditis	- petechiae - **Osler's nodes, Janeway lesions** - indwelling catheters - intravenous drug abuse
toxic shock syndrome	- **erythroderma** (sunburn-appearance) - hands and feet - young females

9.5.) <u>DRUGS OF CHOICE</u>

Actinomyces	actinomycosis	penicillin G
Bacillus anthracis	anthrax	penicillin G
Bordetella pertussis	whooping cough	erythromycin
Borrelia Burgdorferi	Lyme disease	tetracycline
Campylobacter	acute inflammatory diarrhoea	quinolones
Candida	candidiasis	fluconazole
Chlamydia	Pneumonia	tetracycline
	lymphgranuloma venerum	doxycycline
H. influenza	pneumonia, meningitis	3rd gen. Cephalosporin
Helicobacter pylori	gastric ulcer	metronidazole + tetracycline
Klebsiella	Pneumonia	3rd gen. Cephalosporin
	UTI	quinolones
		trimethoprim/sulfamethoxazole
Legionella	Legionnaire's disease	erythromycin
M. tuberculosis	tuberculosis	isoniazide + rifampin
		("2nd line" : cycloserine)
M. leprae	leprosy	dapsone + rifampin
M. pneumoniae	atypical pneumonia	erythromycin
N. gonorrhea	gonorrhea	ceftriaxone
N. meningitis	meningitis	penicillin G
Nocardia	pneumonia	trimethoprim/sulfamethoxazole
Proteus	UTI	quinolones
Rickettsia	spotted fever, end. typhus	doxycycline
Salmonella typhi	typhoid fever	trimethoprim/sulfamethoxazole
Shigella	GI infection	trimethoprim/sulfamethoxazole
Staph. Aureus	skin infection	methicillin
	otitis, Sinusitis	amoxicillin-clavulinate
Strept. Pyogenes	pharyngitis, erysipelas	penicillin G or V
Strept. Viridans	endocarditis	penicillin + aminoglycoside
Treponema pallidum	syphilis	penicillin G
Trichomonas	trichomoniasis	metronidazole
Tropheryma whippelii	Whipple's disease	trimethoprim/sulfamethoxazole
Vibrio cholerae	cholera	tetracycline
Yersinia pestis	plague ("black death")	streptomycin

HEMATOLOGY

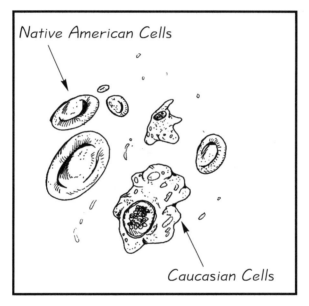

Political Correctness comes to Hematology

10.1.) <u>COAGULATION</u>

bleeding time	- **von Willebrand's** - **thrombocytopenia** - **DIC, ITP, TTP** - **aspirin**
PTT (activated)	- **intrinsic system** (VIII, IX, X, XI, XII) - **heparin** - **hemophilia A and B**
prothrombin time	- **extrinsic system** (VII) - **warfarin** - **vit. K**

INR	- **International Normalized Ratio** to account
	  for variability of thromboplastin preparations.
	
	- calculated from prothrombin time
	- benefits patients who travel,
	  clinical trials, scientific publications

thrombin time	- **heparin** - DIC

 Prolonged use of a tourniquet before drawing blood sample may falsely increase PTT and PT !

10.2.) <u>BLEEDING DISORDERS</u>

coagulation defect	- bleeding into **joints, muscle, viscera** - mainly males
platelet defect	- bleeding into **skin and mucous membranes** - males and females
vascular defect	- **purpura** - gastrointestinal bleeding - mainly females

> _**Von Willebrand's disease**_ :
> - _most common inherited bleeding disorder_
> - _at least 20 subtypes_
> - _autosomal dominant with incomplete penetrance_
> - _prolonged bleeding time and prolonged PTT_

10.3.) <u>HEMOPHILIA</u>

hemophilia A	**- factor VIII deficient** - X-linked recessive - PT normal **- PTT prolonged** - bleeding time normal
hemophilia B	**- factor IX deficient** - X-linked recessive - PT normal **- PTT prolonged** - bleeding time normal
von Willebrand's	**- vWF : qualitative or quantitative dysfunction** - autosomal recessive or dominant - PT normal **- PTT prolonged** **- bleeding time prolonged**

10.4.) <u>BLOOD PRODUCTS</u>

<u>Risk of</u>:

	hepatitis	AIDS	thrombosis
plasma	+	+	-
cryoprecipitate	+	+	-
VIII or IX concentrate	-	-	-
prothrombin complex [1]	++	++	++

[1] rich in factor IX and less expensive than concentrate.

10.5.) <u>HYPERCOAGULABILITY</u>

DIC	- **consumption of coagulation factors** **due to intravascular activation of cascade** - PT prolonged - PTT prolonged - thrombocytopenia - decreased fibrinogen - increased fibrin split products **secondary to** - gram negative sepsis - adenocarcinomas - crash injury - amniotic fluid embolism
antithrombin III	- inhibitor of proteases - blocks thrombin and factor X - potentiates heparin **antithrombin III deficiency (e.g. nephrotic syndrome)** - thrombosis in young adults - *apparent resistance to heparin* !
thrombomodulin	- receptor for thrombin on endothelial cells - thrombin bound to thrombomodulin activates protein C
protein C	- "the body's natural anticoagulant" - inactivates factor V and VIII - stimulates fibrinolysis - vit. K dependent
protein S	- cofactor required for activation of protein C - vit. K dependent
C or S deficiency	- thrombosis in young adults - *oral anticoagulation may result in skin necrosis unless* *heparin is given first !*

10.6.) <u>RED BLOOD CELLS - 1</u>

hematocrit	- normal value in <u>acute</u> blood loss ! - may be false low if blood obtained with capillary fingerstick ("milking")
hemoglobin	- male adult 14-16 g/dl - female adult 12-15 g/dl - newborn 15-25 g/dl
MCH	**MCH (pg) = hemoglobin (g/dL) x 10 / RBC (10^6/μL)**
MCHC	**MCHC (g/dl) = hemoglobin (g/dL) / hematocrit**

↑	**hyperchromatic**
	  - severe dehydration
	  - spherocytosis

↓	**hypochromatic**
	  - overhydration
	  - iron deficiency anemia
	  - thalassemia
	  - sideroblastic anemia

MCV	**MCV (fL) = hematocrit x 1000 / RBC (10^6/μL)**

↑	**macrocytic**
	  - vit B12 deficiency
	  - folate deficiency

↓	**microcytic**
	  - iron deficiency
	  - thalassemia
	  - sideroblastic anemia

10.7.) <u>RED BLOOD CELLS - 2</u>

reticulocyte count	- **percent** of RBCs
reticulocyte count (corrected for hematocrit)	- **percent x (patients HC/ normal HC)** - indicator of erythropoietic activity - if low in an anemic patient suggests chronic disease, deficiency state or marrow suppression.
sedimentation rate	- nonspecific test - infections, inflammations, neoplasms - **increased in anemia !**
direct Coombs' test	- test for **antibodies on patient's erythrocytes** - hemolytic transfusion reaction (mismatch) - autoimmune hemolytic anemia - erythroblastosis fetalis
indirect Coombs' test	- test for **antibodies in patient's serum** - isoimmunization from previous transfusion - Rh sensitization from previous pregnancy
cold agglutinins [1] (antibodies against RBCs)	- mycoplasma pneumonia - mononucleosis - measles, mumps

[1] *don't confuse these with* **cryoglobulins** *= nonspecific immunoglobulins which reversibly precipitate in the cold (multiple myeloma, Waldenström's, lymphoma).*

10.8.) <u>POLYCYTHEMIA</u>

0. RELATIVE	**- RBC mass normal** - plasma volume reduced
1. PRIMARY **polycythemia vera**	**- arises from a single stem cell** - erythrocytosis (elevated RBC mass) - leukocytosis - thrombocytosis - splenomegaly - may convert to AML - *major cause of death: thrombosis !*

2. SECONDARY
 	
 a) COPD
   other lung diseases
   high altitude
	- hypoxemia -> elevated erythropoietin

b) smoker's polycythemia	**- elevated carboxyhemoglobin** - hypoxemia -> elevated erythropoietin

c) kidney diseases
   renal cell carcinoma
   liver cell carcinoma
	- normal blood oxygen saturation
	- elevated erythropoietin

10.9.) <u>MICROCYTIC ANEMIAS</u>

	iron	TIBC	ferritin	comment
chronic disease	↓	↓	↑	
iron deficiency	↓	↑	↓	
thalassemia	∅	∅	∅	- target cells
sideroblastic anemia	↑	∅	↑	
microangiopathic anemia	∅	∅	∅	- helmet cells - schistocytes

10.10.) <u>NORMOCYTIC ANEMIAS</u>

hemolysis	- increased reticulocyte count - increased indirect bilirubin - *do osmotic fragility test* - *do Coombs' test*
chronic renal failure	- burr cells

10.11.) <u>MACROCYTIC ANEMIAS</u>

vit. B12 deficiency **folate deficiency**	- normochromic RBCs - hypersegmented neutrophils (band forms)
aplastic anemia	- normochromic RBCs - hypocellular marrow - pancytopenia

	folic acid	vit. B12
alcoholics	↓	↓
phenytoin	↓	-
strict vegetarians	-	↓
strict vegetable avoiders	↓	-

10.12.) <u>SICKLE CELL ANEMIAS</u>

SA - sickle cell trait	**- 60% HbA** **- 40% HbS** - asymptomatic - prevalence 10% in African-American population
SS - sickle cell anemia	**- 90% HbS** **- 10% HbF** - severe anemia - sickle cell crisis (microinfarction of vital organs) - auto-splenectomy
SC - disease	**- 50% HbS** **- 50% HbC** - moderate anemia - may become severe during pregnancy !

HbC contains a point mutation on the β-chain at the same amino acid position as the HbS.mutation.

10.13.) <u>THALASSEMIAS</u>

thalassemia minor (heterozygote)	- 90% HbA - 5% HbA_2 - 5% HbF - mild anemia - may be asymptomatic
thalassemia major (homozygote)	- 5% HbA_2 - 95% HbF - severe anemia - requires transfusions - iron overload
α-carrier (deletion of 1 α gene)	- asymptomatic
α-trait (deletion of 2 α genes)	- asymptomatic - microcytic hypochrome RBCs
HbH disease (deletion of 3 α genes)	- 70% HbA - 30% HbH - mild to moderate anemia - microcytic hypochrome RBCs
homozygous α thalassemia (deletion of 4 α genes)	**- only HbH and Hb Bart** - hydrops fetalis (stillbirth)

$$HbA_2 = \alpha_2\delta_2 \,, \ HbF = \alpha_2\gamma_2 \,, \ HbH = \beta_4 \,, \ Hb\ Bart = \gamma_4$$

10.14.) <u>AUTOIMMUNE HEMOLYTIC ANEMIAS</u>

warm type	cold type
usually IgG	**usually IgM**
- lymphoma, CLL	- mononucleosis
- SLE	- mycoplasma infection
- viral infections	- lymphoma
- drugs : **penicillin**	
quinidine	

<u>*Two unusual but interesting diseases:*</u>

Paroxysmal nocturnal hemolytic disease:
- RBCs, granulocytes and platelets are unusually sensitive to complement.
- Coombs' test negative.
- RBC lysis occurs in hypotonic solution (sugar water test).

Paroxysmal cold hemoglobinuria:
- IgG against red blood cell P-antigen binds in the cold.
- complement mediated RBC lysis occurs after rewarming blood.
  (Donath-Landsteiner antibodies)

10.15.) <u>WHITE BLOOD CELLS</u>

	increased	decreased

neutrophils	- **bacterial infections**
	- inflammation
	- exercise, stress
	- pregnancy
	- corticosteroids
		- **bone marrow suppression**
		  cytotoxic drugs
		  chloramphenicol
		  chlorpromazine
		  quinine
		
		- **overwhelming infections**
		  (disseminated TB, sepsis)

eosinophils	- **allergy** - **parasites**	- steroids - stress
lymphocytes	- **viral infections** - ALL - CLL	- stress - bone marrow suppression - AIDS
platelets	- exercise - splenectomy	- **DIC** - **ITP** - **TTP**

 atypical lymphocytes : *infectious mononucleosis*

 "Left shift" : *bacterial infection, hemorrhage*
"Right shift" : *megaloblastic anemia, iron deficiency anemia*

10.16.) LEUKEMIAS

	ALL (3-7 years) [1]	AML (all ages)	CML (50 years)	CLL (70 years)	Hairy cells (50 years)
	fever petechiae ecchymoses CNS infiltrate	fever petechiae ecchymoses lymphadenopathy (splenomegaly)	fever night sweats splenomegaly	insidious few symptoms low Ig levels infections	hepatomegaly splenomegaly TRAP
prognosis	prognosis : fair	poor	poor	fair	poor
	lymphoblasts	Auer rods in myeloblasts a/w irradiation chemotherapy	Philadelphia chr. in myeloid stem cells: t(9q;22q)	lymphocytes predominate	pancytopenia hairy cells in bone marrow

[1] median age of onset.

161

10.17.) THROMBOCYTOPENIA

- < 100,000/μl increased bleeding risk
- < 20,000/μl spontaneous bleeding
- < 10,000/μl CNS bleeding

megakaryocyte depression	- viral infections - drugs
general bone marrow failure	- myelophtisis - radiation
platelet destruction	- ITP
platelet consumption	- TTP - DIC
platelet sequestration	- splenomegaly

ITP	TTP
- immune mediated destruction of platelets - increased number of bone marrow megakaryocytes **in children** - often follows viral infections - resolves spontaneously **in adults** - unknown cause - more chronic	1. thrombocytopenia 2. microthrombi -> hemolytic anemia (helmet cells) 3. neurological symptoms 4. fever 5. mild azotemia **- affects mainly young women**

 Hemolytic uremic syndrome resembles TTP, except that it affects primarily the kidneys (acute renal failure, no neurological symptoms).

10.18.) <u>SPLENOMEGALY</u>

mild	- infections - right heart failure
moderate	- acute leukemias - lymphomas - hemolytic anemias - infectious mononucleosis - liver cirrhosis / hepatitis
massive	- CML - myelofibrosis - thalassemia major - Gaucher's / Niemann-Pick

10.19.) <u>HODGKIN'S DISEASE</u>

Stage I	- single lymph node
Stage II	- two or more lymph nodes on same side of diaphragm
Stage III	- lymph nodes on both sides of diaphragm
Stage IV	- diffuse involvement of extralymphatic sites

> **A:** *Constitutional symptoms absent*
> **B:** *Constitutional symptoms present*

 Staging laparoscopy only if anticipated therapeutic consequence. Example: If patient has clinical Stage III or IV, staging operation is unnecessary since treatment is chemotherapy anyway.

Hodgkin's Disease	**Non-Hodgkin Lymphomas**
- spreads in contiguity - no leukemic component - Reed-Sternberg cells	- do not spread in contiguity - often have leukemic component

Hot-List

BLEEDING DISORDERS

Hemophilia
- avoid trauma
- never use aspirin
- heat-treated factor VIII (hemophilia A) or IX (hemophilia B) concentrate

Von Willebrand's
- for mild disease: no treatment necessary, but avoid aspirin
- standard therapy: cryoprecipitate (danger of hepatitis and HIV transmission)
- new factor VIII concentrates may become available that contain vWF and do not transmit hepatitis or HIV

PLATELET DISORDERS

DIC
- identify and treat underlying disorder
- replacement: platelet transfusions, cryoprecipitate (platelets)
- heparin is controversial: may be necessary if underlying cause cannot be identified, but may induce unacceptable bleeding

TTP
- emergency large-volume plasmapheresis
- splenectomy if non-responsive

ITP
- prednisone decreases affinity of splenic macrophages for antibody coated platelets
- splenectomy is definite treatment

Hemolytic-Uremic Syndrome
- in children almost always self-limited
- in adults 80% rate of chronic renal failure if untreated
  (requires large-volume plasmapheresis)

RED BLOOD CELL DISORDERS

Sickle Cell Anemia
- folic acid supplementation
- transfusions indicated for aplastic or hemolytic crisis
- exchange transfusion for acute vaso-occlusive crisis

Thalassemia
- α-trait or β-minor : no therapy necessary
- give folate supplements. It's a microcytic anemia, but avoid iron !
- severe anemia: maintain regular transfusion schedule
- deferoxamine (iron-chelator)
- β-major: consider bone marrow transplantation

Polycythemia Vera
- phlebotomy
- myelosuppression if excessive platelet count (thrombosis risk)
- avoid alkylating agents or ^{32}P: increased risk of acute leukemia
- allopurinol for hyperuricemia

WHITE BLOOD CELL DISORDERS

Agranulocytosis
- hospitalize
- prompt wide-spectrum antibiotic cover

Acute Leukemias
- young patients - goal is effective cure
- combination chemotherapy
- remission induction for ALL is less myelosuppressive than for AML
- consider bone marrow transplantation
- after remission: CNS prophylaxis: radiation and intrathecal methotrexate

CLL

- most indolent cases don't require specific therapy
- chlorambucil or prednisone for progressive fatigue and lymphadenopathy

CML

- **palliative**: continuous hydroxyurea to suppress white blood cell count
- good response to α-interferon (dramatically reduces number of Philadelphia chromosome positive cells)
- **curative**: allogenic bone marrow transplantation (from HLA-matched siblings). Success rate 60-80% if performed early

Hodgkin's Disease

- if localized: radiation
- if disseminated: aggressive combination chemotherapy

Non-Hodgkin's Lymphoma

- combination chemotherapy
- Regimen and therapeutic intent (palliative vs. curative) depends on disease stage and histology

Waldenström's

- plasmapheresis to reduce blood hyperviscosity
- intermittent chemotherapy (chlorambucil, cyclophosphamide) if necessary

Multiple Myeloma

- goal of treatment usually palliative
- combination chemotherapy
- localized radiotherapy for bone pain
- allogenic bone marrow transplantation (from HLA-matched siblings) is promising

ENDOCRINE
DISEASES

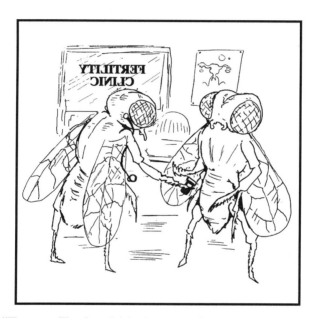

"These pills should help, Mrs. Gordon, but you
might lay up to 20,000 eggs."

11.1.) <u>ANTERIOR PITUITARY</u>
(Hypofunction)

FSH and LH ↓	- **early sign of pituitary failure** - irregular menstruation - amenorrhea
ACTH ↓	**similar to Addison's disease** - weakness - malaise - nausea, vomiting - <u>but no hyperpigmentation</u> !
TSH ↓	- depression - apathy

Sheehan's syndrome:
Hypofunction due to postpartum hemorrhage.

11.2.) <u>ANTERIOR PITUITARY</u>
(Hyperfunction)

prolactin ↑	**in women:** - galactorrhea - amenorrhea **in men:** - impotence, loss of libido - galactorrhea
GH ↑	- **children**: giantism - **adults**: enlarged jaw, forehead, hands and feet - reduced glucose tolerance - osteoarthritis
ACTH ↑	- signs of excess glucocorticoids - signs of excess mineralocorticoids - <u>high dose</u> dexamethasone suppresses cortisol levels

 Usually adenomas, very rarely carcinomas.

<u>Causes of prolactinemia:</u>

physiologic	- pregnancy - lactation - nipple stimulation
pathologic	- prolactinomas - craniopharyngiomas - empty sella syndrome
drugs	- phenothiazines - methyldopa - reserpine

 Prolactin secretion is under chronic inhibitory control of dopamine.

11.3.) <u>POSTERIOR PITUITARY</u>

<u>Hypofunction:</u>

	result of overnight water deprivation
central diabetes insipidus (lack of ADH secretion)	- urine osmolarity increases >50% after injection of vasopressin (ADH)
renal diabetes insipidus (lack of ADH responsiveness**)**	- urine osmolarity increases little after injection of vasopressin (ADH)
primary polydipsia (psychogenic)	- urine osmolarity >> plasma osmolarity

<u>Hyperfunction:</u>   **Inappropriate Secretion of ADH**

signs of SIADH	- hypotonic volume expansion - renal sodium wasting
causes of SIADH	- **CNS disease**: trauma, tumors, infections - **ectopic malignancies**: lymphomas, leukemias, bronchial carcinomas - **pulmonary disease**: pneumonia, tbc, PEEP - **drugs**: carbamazepine, tricyclic antidepressants, MAO inhibitors....

11.4.) ADRENAL GLAND

Cushing's syndrome	**excess glucocorticoids**
	- truncal obesity
	- moon face
	- buffalo hump
	- osteoporosis
	- skin atrophy (striae)
	- virilization, amenorrhea
	
	- failure of low dose dexamethasone suppression
	  confirms Cushing's syndrome.
	- high dose suppression test distinguishes between
	  Cushing's disease and adenoma.

Conn's syndrome	**primary hyperaldosteronism (signs)** - sodium retention - hypertension - potassium loss **secondary hyperaldosteronism (causes)** - congestive heart failure - liver cirrhosis - nephrotic syndrome
Addison's disease	**primary corticoadrenal insufficiency** **deficiency of mineralocorticoids** - sodium loss, hyperkalemia - metabolic acidosis **deficiency of glucocorticoids** - anorexia, weight loss, apathy - stress intolerance **high ACTH and MSH** - characteristic pigmentation of skin folds

Addisonian crisis :
Minor stress or illness may cause fever, shock and
coma due to lack of glucocorticoids.

11.5.) <u>GLUCOCORTICOIDS</u>

increased	- Cushing's disease - adrenal adenoma - adrenal carcinoma
decreased	- Addison's disease - Waterhouse-Friderichsen - congenital adrenal hyperplasia

---

Dexamethasone suppression should suppress plasma cortisol < 5 µg/dl

---

overnight test	- failure to suppress **suggests Cushing's syndrome**
	
	- false positive: obesity
	                    alcoholism
	                    depression

low dose test (48h)	- failure to suppress **confirms Cushing's syndrome**
high dose test (48h)	- *do if low dose fails to suppress cortisol* - if cortisol < 5 µg/dl : **Cushing's disease** - if cortisol > 5 µg/dl : **adrenal tumor** or **ectopic ACTH**

Cushing's syndrome : *Cortisol excess*
Cushing's disease   : *Pituatary ACTH -> Cortisol excess*

11.6.) <u>URINARY METABOLITES</u>

17-hydroxycorticosteroids	- Cushing's - adrenogenital syndrome
17-ketosteroids	- androstenedione and DHEA - pituitary, adrenal or testicular tumors
vanillylmandelic acid, metanephrines	- catecholamines : **pheochromocytoma**
5-hydroxyindoleacetic acid	- serotonin metabolite : **carcinoid**

11.7.) __THYROID HORMONES__

T3, T4	- **increased** : hyperthyroidism estrogens, pregnancy - **decreased** : euthyroid sick state hypothyroidism
T3 resin uptake	- **increased** : hyperthyroidism nephrotic syndrome (TBG $\downarrow$) steroids, heparin, aspirin, others - **decreased** : hypothyroidism estrogens, pregnancy (TBG$\uparrow$)
TSH	- **increased** : primary hypothyroidism (Hashimoto's) pituitary adenoma - **decreased** : primary hyperthyroidism (Graves') pituitary insufficiency

NORMAL   HYPOTHYROIDISM   PREGNANCY

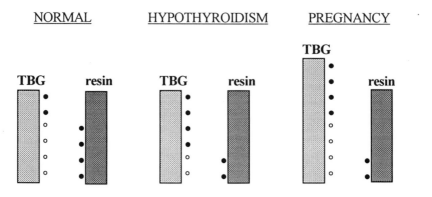

$\circ$ T_3
$\bullet$ T_3 (radiolabeled)
number of $\bullet$ on resin = T_3 resin uptake

11.8.) <u>THYROID GLAND</u>

hyperthyroidism	hypothyroidism
- heat intolerance - nervousness - palpitations, atrial fibrillation - weight loss (good appetite !)	- cold intolerance - constipation - coarse hair - myxedema - weight gain (low appetite !)

- <u>most common cause:</u>
  Graves' disease
	- <u>most common cause:</u>
	  Hashimoto's thyroiditis

Graves' disease	- antibodies to TSH receptors stimulate thyroid - radioactive iodine uptake very high - exophtalmus - <u>pretibial</u> myxedema [1]
congenital hypothyroidism	- cretinism - iodine deficiency or thyroid dysgenesis
acquired hypothyroidism	- Hashimoto's thyroiditis (autoimmune) - patient's treated previously for hyper- thyroidism with ^{131}I
sick euthyroid syndrome	- T3 and T4 low - TSH normal - no clinical signs of hypothyroidism !

[1] do not confuse with myxedema of hypothyroidism !

11.9.) <u>GLUCOSE</u>

fasting glucose	- **blood**: 60 -100 mg/dl - **plasma**: 70-110 mg/dl
oral glucose tolerance	- perform if fasting glucose 110-140 mg/ml - pregnancy screening ("glucola")

<u>Diabetes mellitus</u>:
fasting plasma glucose > 140 mg/ml (two occasions)
or 1h and 2h values > 200 mg/ml

<u>Impaired glucose tolerance</u>:
fasting plasma glucose < 140 mg/ml
and 2h value 140-200 mg/ml
and at least one intervening value > 200 mg/d

11.10.) <u>DIABETES MELLITUS</u>

	IDDM	NIDDM
onset	juvenile	adult
body weight	normal	obese
ketoacidosis	common	rare
insulin resistance	rare	almost always
identical twin concordance	< 50%	almost 100%
HLA association	DR3, DR4	none
other autoimmune diseases	associated	not associated

insulin RIA	- to diagnose insulinoma or islet cell hyperplasia
insulin, C-peptide	- if patient is hypoglycemic and C-peptide is not elevated: suspect factitious disorder !

Hot-List

PITUITARY

Sheehan's
- hydrocortisone
- levothyroxine
- estrogens
- induction of ovulation: clomiphene

Acromegaly
- bone growth is irreversible
- transphenoidal resection or supervoltage radiation
- follow patient for signs of hypopituitarism

Diabetes Insipidus
- if central: intranasal desmopressin
- if renal: thiazides !

SIADH
- saline (3%) plus furosemide (prevents kidneys to excrete extra sodium)
- correct sodium levels slowly (danger of central pontine demyelination)

ADRENAL

Cushing's
- do high dose dexamethasone suppression test if low dose test confirms Cushing's syndrome
- remove pituitary tumor or ectopic tumor
- if ACTH comes from widespread metastases suppress adrenal cortisol secretion with ketoconazole or metyrapone

Addison's Crisis

- obtain plasma sample to determine ACTH
- perform rapid ACTH stimulation test if possible
- administer IV hydrocortisone
- correct fluid and electrolytes, watch K^+
- lifelong supplementation with glucocorticoids (e.g. hydrocortisone) and mineralocorticoids (e.g. fludrocortisone)

Pheochromocytoma

- localize with ^{131}I-metaiodobenzylguanidine scan
- α-blockade before surgical removal

THYROID

Hyperthyroidism (Graves')

- ^{131}I (risk of hypothyroidism after 10 years: 70%)
- surgical ablation (risk of hypothyroidism after 10 years: 40%)
- propylthiouracil is drug of choice during pregnancy

Thyrotoxic Crisis

- propylthiouracil
- propranolol
- iodide

Hypothyroidism

- L-thyroxine

Thyroid Cancer

- total thyroidectomy - followed by ^{131}I except medullary carcinoma (C cells)

METABOLISM

Hyperlipidemia
- rule out secondary causes (hypothyroidism, diabetes, alcohol abuse, β-blockers, corticosteroids, thiazides)
- weight reduction: diet, exercise
- calculate LDL for patient monitoring. If diet fails, consider drug therapy
- there is no "ideal" cholesterol. The more risk factors for CAD are present, the more aggressively should cholesterol be lowered
- **high triglycerides**: fibrates and nicotinic acid
- **high LDL cholesterol**: bile acid sequestrants, HMG CoA reductase inhibitors, niacin

IDDM
- regular meal times and caloric content
- adjust insulin types and times according to daily glucose profile
- nocturnal hypoglycemia may result in morning hyperglycemia ! You should decrease the insulin dose !
- home blood glucose monitoring
- glycosylated hemoglobin (HbA_{1C}) to assess long term control. Not useful for specific adjustments to insulin therapy

NIDDM
- weight loss is most important
- sulfonylureas
- if insulin necessary see above

MUSCULOSKELETAL DISEASES

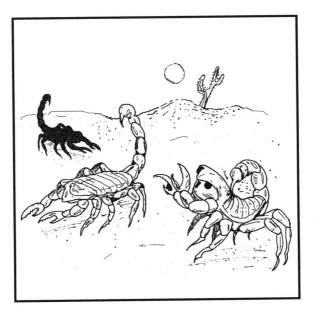

**Lumbar spinal lordosis – major killer of
the desert scorpion.**

12.1.) <u>AUTOANTIBODIES</u>

ANA	- **sensitive** but not specific for SLE *(for screening !)*
ds-DNA	- **specific** but not sensitive for SLE *(for workup !)* - correlates with disease activity
Sm [1]	- **specific** but not sensitive for SLE
anti-histone	- drug induced SLE

[1] *don't confuse with anti smooth muscle antibodies (sclerosing cholangitis)*

anti-centromere	- specific and sensitive for CREST
anti-Scl 70	- specific but not sensitive for systemic sclerosis
anti-SS-A (Ro)	- Sjögren's syndrome
anti-SS-B (La)	- Sjögren's syndrome - less frequent than Ro
c-ANCA	- Wegener's granulomatosis
p-ANCA	- less sensitive and specific than c-ANCA
rheumatoid factor	- (auto-antibodies against IgG) - sensitive but not specific for rheumatoid arthritis - tends to correlate with disease severity

ANA : *ds-DNA, ss-DNA, histones*
ENA : *(soluble nonhistone proteins): Sm, Ro, La*

12.2.) <u>BONES AND MINERALS</u>

	Ca^{2+}	phosphate	alk. phosphatase	PTH
hypoparathyroidism	↓	↑	O	↓
pseudohypoparathyroidism	↓	↑	O	↑
osteoporosis	O	O	O	O
osteomalacia	↓	↓	↑	↑
Vit. D intoxication	↑	↑	O	↓

185

12.3.) <u>ARTHRITIS</u>

rheumatoid arthritis	osteoarthritis
autoimmune disease	**degenerative disease**
- morning stiffness - swelling of 3 or more joints	- progressive pain - relieved by rest
- ***wrist, MCP and PIP involved*** - subcutaneous nodules	- hip joint, knee joint - ***DIP and PIP (in women !)***
- rheumatoid factor - HLA-DR1 and DR4	
<u>x-ray</u> - joint erosions - periarticular bone erosions	<u>x-ray</u> - loss of cartilage - narrowed joint space - subchondral cysts and sclerosis - new bone formation (marginal osteophytes)
characteristic hand deformity **"swan neck"** - metacarpophalangeal subluxation - ulnar deviation of digits - hyperextension of PIP	

<u>Systemic manifestations of</u>
<u>rheumatoid arthritis:</u>
- *rheumatoid nodules*
- *uveitis, retinitis*
- *pleuritis*
- *pericarditis*
- *myocarditis*
- *vasculitis*

12.4.) <u>GOUT</u>

gout	pseudogout
- **urate** crystals - severe but self limited pain attack	- **calcium pyrophosphate** crystals - attack resembles gout - chronic phase resembles RA
- first metatarsal joint	- often involves knee joint
- **strongly negative birefringent crystals (needle shaped, yellow)**	- **weakly positive birefringent crystals (rhomboid, blue)**
- *aspirin is contraindicated*	

<u>*Charcot joint:*</u>
 - *loss of proprioception (tabes, diabetic neuropathy...)*
 - *repeat trauma*
 - *joint instability, swelling*
 - *painless*

12.5.) <u>SYNOVIAL EFFUSIONS</u>

	appearance	WBC / µl
normal	- colorless to straw-colored	< 200 < 25% PMN
<u>**non-inflammatory**</u> osteoarthritis trauma	- straw-colored	< 2000 30% PMN
<u>**inflammatory**</u> SLE gout pseudogout rheumatoid arthritis	- yellow	> 2000 75% PMN
<u>**septic**</u> bacterial infections	- yellow and cloudy - gram stain !	> 100.000 > 75% PMN

<u>**Gonococcal arthritis**</u>:
- young adults
- "migratory joint pain"
- eventually settles in 1 or 2 joints

12.6.) <u>SPONDYLOARTHROPATHIES</u>

- **involve sacroiliac joint**
  (destruction of cartilage, subchondral erosions, pseudo-widening)
- **seronegative for rheumatoid factor**

ankylosing spondylitis	- more common in young men - gradual onset - a/w HLA-B27 - **always sacroilitis**
Reiter's syndrome (reactive arthritis)	- more common in men - sudden onset - a/w HLA-B27 - **urethritis** - **arthritis (knees, ankle)** - postdysenteric (shigella) - postveneral (chlamydia)
psoriatic arthritis	- more common in women - variable onset - occurs in 20% of psoriatic patients - weakly a/w HLA-B27 - nail pitting - sausage toes

12.7.) ADOLESCENT'S OSTEOCHONDROSES

Osgood-Schlatter	Legg-Calvé-Perthes	Scheuermann's
- **osteochondritis of tibia tubercle**	- **slipped capital femoral epiphysis** (aseptic necrosis)	- **vertebral osteochondritis**
- pain and swelling of tubercle - following trauma or exercise - usually unilateral - more common in boys	- develops slowly - usually unilateral - more common in obese boys - hip pain referred to thigh or knee	- "round shouldered posture" - persistent lowgrade backache - thoracic kyphosis - male > female
- **x-ray**: calcified thickening irregular ossification	- **x-ray**: flattening and fragmentation of femoral head	- **x-ray**: anterior wedging of vertebrae
- *resolves spontaneously* - *avoid exercise (knee bends)* - *if persistent: steroids*	- *bed rest* - *mobile traction* - *splints* - *if untreated predisposes to osteoarthritis*	- *avoid weightbearing stress* - *rest on rigid bed* - *surgical correction in severe cases*

12.8.) LUPUS

systemic lupus	- **butterfly rash (spares nasolabial fold)** - **discoid rash** - arthritis - serositis - nephrotic syndrome - anemia - leukopenia, lymphopenia - thrombocytopenia - antinuclear antibodies - false positive serology for syphilis (anticardiolipin antibodies)
discoid lupus (5-10% -> SLE)	- disease limited to skin: - **scaly lesions with raised erythematous rim** - **leave disfiguring scars** - patchy loss of scalp hair (irreversible)
subacute cutaneous lupus	- **wide-spread annular, nonscarring lesions** - **photosensitivity** - often ANA negative - anti-Ro positive
drug induced lupus	- often mild - **reversible** after drug cessation - ANA may persist for years

---

> ***Common drugs that may induce lupus :***
> - *hydralazine*
> - *procainamide*
> - *isoniazid*
> - *chlorpromazine*
> - *methyldopa...*

12.9.) <u>SCLERODERMA</u>

localized scleroderma = morphea	- more common in children - violet, expanding lesions - may be disfiguring if on forehead ("coup de sabre")
limited systemic sclerosis = CREST	- Calcinosis - Raynaud's - Esophageal dysmotility - Sclerodactyly - Telangiectasia - rarely involves internal organs - fair prognosis - **anti-centromere antibody**
progressive systemic sclerosis	- like CREST, but more rapid progression of skin disease and early involvement of internal organs. **renal crisis** - malignant hypertension - oliguria **pulmonary disease** - interstitial fibrosis - poor prognosis - **anti-topoisomerase antibody** (Scl-70)

 Raynaud's phenomenon is often the earliest symptom.

12.10.) <u>INFLAMMATORY MYOPATHIES</u>

- slowly progressive, symmetric proximal muscle weakness
- elevated muscle enzymes (creatine kinase, aldolase)
- biopsy: lymphocytic inflammation

- 20% associated with autoimmune diseases: RA, SLE, SS
- 10% associated with malignancies: lung, breast, ovary, colon...

dermatomyositis	polymyositis
- myopathy	- myopathy
- heliotrope rash (purple discoloration of upper eye lids) - facial rash (resembles lupus but involves nasolabial fold) - rash of V-region of neck - erythema of knuckles, knees, elbows	- no rash - no calcinosis
- calcinosis	

Polymyalgia rheumatica: *- proximal muscle weakness*
- serum CPK normal

193

12.11.) <u>VASCULITIS</u>

hypersensitivity [1]	**- small vessels** - lesions all at same stage - cryoglobulins
polyarteritis nodosa	**- small and medium vessels** - kidney, heart, GI tract - does not affect lung
giant cell arteritis	**- temporal artery** - sudden blindness ! - female > male - very high ESR - a/w polymyalgia rheumatica
Wegener's	**- upper respiratory vasculitis** **- lower respiratory vasculitis** - glomerulonephritis
Takayasu	**- aorta / large arteries** - "pulseless disease" (upper extremity claudication) - Asian females
Kawasaki	- mucocutaneous lymph node syndrome - fever, conjunctivitis, maculopapular rash **- coronary artery aneurysms** - Japanese children

[1] *Example:* ***Henoch Schönlein****: - purpura (buttocks)*
- abdominal pain
- arthritis
- hematuria

Hot-List

Osteoarthritis
- exercise, physical therapy
- if knee joints involved: diet and weight loss
- NSAIDs. Acetaminophen less toxic than salicylates

Rheumatoid Arthritis
- aspirin, other NSAIDs. Consider misoprostol to reduce gastric ulceration
- methotraxate for severe cases. Used in much lower dosage than for anti-tumor therapy
- gold, penicillamine, quinine: Don't expect beneficial effect until 2-6 months after initiating therapy

Gout
- do not treat asymptomatic hyperuricemia
- **acute attack**: treat acute arthritis first, hyperuricemia later. Sudden reduction of uric acid may precipitate further attacks !
- NSAIDs except aspirin
- colchicine (may cause severe stomach cramps)
- **between attacks**: diet (avoid meat, kidney, liver, alcohol). Avoid aspirin.
- uricosuric drugs: maintain good urinary output
- allopurinol: for patients with uric acid overproduction

Pseudogout
- NSAIDs
- colchicine is less effective for acute attack of pseudogout than it is for gout

Ankylosing Spondylitis
- physical therapy. Postural exercises. Breathing exercises
- NSAIDs. Indomethacin especially effective
- 10% of patients will have work disability after 10 years

SLE
- benign cases require only supportive care and emotional support
- NSAIDs for joint symptoms - antimalarials (hydoxychloroquinine) if unresponsive
- topical corticosteroids for skin lesions. Avoid sun exposure (photosensitivity)
- systemic corticosteroids for serious complications: TTP, myocarditis, nephritis etc.
- if resistant to steroids try immunosuppressants (cyclophosphamide, azathioprine...)
- thrombosis in young women: think 1.) oral contraceptives, 2.) SLE (antiphospholipid antibodies). Requires oral anticoagulation

Dermatomyositis
- corticosteroids
- taper slowly and monitor muscle enzymes
- IV immunoglobulin if unresponsive to steroids
- search for underlying malignancies. These may not become apparent for months after onset of dermatomyositis

Rickets
- Vitamin D
- if resistant to Vit. D (rare renal tubular defect): give phosphate and Vit. D_3

Paget's Disease
- (osteitis deformans)
- synthetic salmon calcitonin suppresses osteoclastic activity
- human calcitonin is more expensive but less allergenic
- watch for renal complications secondary to hypercalciuria !

Osteomyelitis
- aspirate and culture to select antibiotic
- immobilization
- IV antibiotics, followed by oral for 6 weeks after fever normalized
- surgical debridement for refractory cases

Carpal Tunnel Syndrome
- relief of pressure on median nerve: hand elevation, splinting of hand and forearm, injection of corticosteroids into carpal tunnel
- surgical separation of volar carpal ligament gives lasting relief

DISEASES
OF THE
EYES AND SKIN

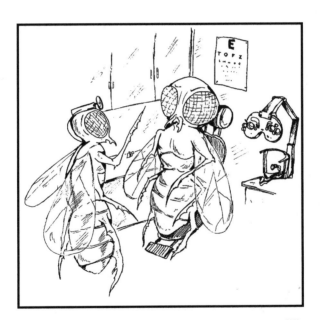

**"Now how many fingers do you see, one million
or two million?"**

13.1.) <u>RED EYE</u>

conjunctivitis	- most commonly viral (highly contagious) - eyelids "stuck together" in the morning - mucoid discharge - usually not painful
uveitis	- hazy vision - perilimbal injection
subconjunctival hemorrhage	- following increased intrathoracic pressure (coughing, sneezing, Valsalva) - will resolve spontaneously - **painless**
cornea abrasion	- result of minor trauma - "foreign body sensation" - diagnosis: fluorescein dye - **painful** - *prevent bacterial superinfection* !
herpes	- conjunctivitis, scarring - dendritic keratitis - **corneal anesthesia**
acute glaucoma	- dilated pupils - **very painful**

13.2.) <u>CONJUNCTIVITIS</u>

	allergic	bacterial	viral
itching	**severe**	little	little
injection	mild	**severe**	moderate
discharge	mild	**severe**	moderate
preauricular LN	negative	negative	**enlarged**
associated with	hay fever		sore throat
treatment	*steroids antihistamines*	*topical antibiotics*	*preventive*

13.3.) <u>GLAUCOMA</u>

open angle	**- asymptomatic until late stage** - gradual loss of peripheral vision (tunnel vision)
closed angle	**- rapid onset** **- severe pain** - blurred vision - reddened eye - dilated, non-reactive pupils - due to blockage of aqueous drainage - may be precipitated by pupil dilation (atropine)

13.4.) RETINA

hypertensive retinopathy	- "copper wire arterioles" - "cotton wool spots" - vein indentations at a.v. crossings - edematous papilla
diabetic retinopathy	- microaneurysms - new vessel formation - "cotton wool spots"
senile macular degeneration	- **slow painless loss of central visual acuity** - pigment disturbances - exudative mounds - scar formation
retinal detachment	- **painless** - flashes of light, blurred vision - retinal irregularities, breaks and detachments
optic neuritis	- **painful sudden** loss of vision - optic disc swollen - flame shaped hemorrhages
central retinal artery occlusion	- **painless sudden** loss of vision - optic disc pale - cherry red fovea - vessels appear bloodless
central retinal vein occlusion	- **painless gradual** loss of vision - a/w diabetes, glaucoma, high blood viscosity - tortuous, distended veins - numerous retinal hemorrhages

13.5.) DERMATITIS

acute contact dermatitis	"a rash that itches" **irritants** - soap - detergents **allergens** - poison ivy - metals - drugs
atopic dermatitis	"an itch that rashes" - a/w asthma, hay fever - worsened by stress, premenstrual
seborrheic dermatitis	- scaly, oily patches - slight erythema at base - scalp - eye brows - retroauricular - presternal
stasis dermatitis	- venous stasis, thrombophlebitis - deposition of hemosiderin - ulceration - typically just above medial malleolus
lichen simplex	- large, circumscribed scaling patches - skin thickening - results from chronic scratching and rubbing

13.6.) <u>SKIN TUMORS</u>

seborrheic keratosis ("senile warts")	- benign epidermal tumors - very common in the elderly - multiple occurrence - usually pigmented, scaly
actinic keratosis	- scaly red patches on sun exposed areas - may develop into squamous cell carcinoma (risk about 1%)
squamous cell carcinoma	- ulcerated erosion or nodule
keratoacanthoma	- subtype of squamous cell carcinoma - berry like nodule - grows very rapidly
basal cell carcinoma	**nodular type** - translucent, pearly, white appearance - raised borders - may be ulcerated - bleeds easily **superficial type** - scaly red patch - well demarcated
melanoma	<u>compared to simple nevus:</u> - **Asymmetrical** - **Borders irregular, notched** - **Color: various shades of brown** - **Diameter increasing** **Metastases: skin, brain, fetus**

 Avoid UV-B. Use sunscreen, especially at young age !

13.7.) <u>VASCULAR TUMORS</u>

capillary hemangiomas	- malformation of capillaries
	
	nevus flammeus
	  - spontaneous regression
	
	"portwine stain"
	  - form of nevus flammeus that does not regress
	
	"strawberry" hemangiomas
	  - rapid growth for 3-6 months
	  - usually complete regression in one year

cavernous hemangiomas	- malformation of larger blood vessels - superficial: bright, red color - deep ones: bluish color - do not regress spontaneously
Sturge-Weber	**- follows trigeminal distribution** - cutaneous hemangiomas - leptomeningeal hemangiomas - possible degeneration of cerebral cortex (-> seizures, hemiplegia)

13.8.) <u>OTHER SKIN DISEASES</u>

pemphigus	- vesicles on mucosa - **autoantibodies** against intercellular junctions of keratinocytes *TX: hospitalization, systemic corticosteroids* *immunosuppression, plasmapheresis*
pemphigoid	- like pemphigus, but larger bullae on abdomen, groin - more common in the elderly - not life-threatening *TX: systemic corticosteroids*
impetigo	- **honey colored crust**, superficial skin infection - Staph. aureus (or β-hemolytic streptococci) *TX: β-lactamase resistant penicillin or cephalosporin*
pityriasis	- eggshaped, rose colored **herald patch** on trunk - followed by smaller lesions spreading along flexural lines *TX: none, resolves spontaneously*
rosacea	- telangiectasia, erythema, papules and pustules (face and nose) - looks like acne, but no comedones - may result in **nose tissue hypertrophy** (rhinophyma) *TX: metronidazole, wide spectrum antibiotics* *corticosteroids are contraindicated !*
scabies	- parasitic skin infection (mites) - intense itch, **burrows** - spares face *TX: Lindane or Elimite cream.* *Mites don't survive off body*

EYES

Chalazion / Sty
- Chalazion = internal hordeulum (Meibomian gland)
- Stye = external hordeulum (glands of Zeiss or Moll)
- treatment is the same: warm compresses and topical antibiotics

Glaucoma
- **open angle (non-urgent)**
- topical: pilocarpine, β-blockers. Systemic: acetazolamide
- **closed angle (emergency)**
- topical: pilocarpine, β-blockers
- laser iridectomy when eye is quiet

Cataracts
- chronic pupillary dilation may help
- lens extraction (age is no contraindication)
- corticosteroids for uveitis

Diabetic Retinopathy
- annual ophthalmoscopic exam
- sugar control: retards, but does not reverse retinopathy
- photocoagulation diminishes neovascularization

Retinal Detachment
- emergency, even if small (entire retina may detach !)
- hospitalize patient, keep head elevated, eye patches
- urgent surgical reattachment

SKIN

Acne
- benzyl peroxide
- retinoic acid cream, antibiotics
- oral isotretinoin only for severe pustular acne

Contact Dermatitis
- remove offending agent
- antihistamines or desensitization are ineffective
- topical steroids are ineffective in blistering phase (consider systemic if severe)
- topical steroids are effective in dry phase

Seborrhoic Dermatitis
- daily zinc, selenium, sulfur, tar shampoos
- topical hydrocortisone (avoid fluorinated corticosteroids -> skin atrophy)

Psoriasis
- lubrication, keratolysis, topical corticosteroids
- avoid systemic steroids
- PUVA: oral psoralen and ultraviolet A radiation
- for severe disabling cases consider methotrexate

Candidiasis
- oral (trush): nystatin suspension
- cutaneous: nystatin powder
- systemic: oral ketoconazole, fluconazole

Secondary Syphilis
- Penicillin. Watch out for Herxheimer reaction !
- tetracycline or erythromycin if allergic to penicillin

Stasis Ulcer

- leg elevation, compression bandage
- surgical removal of varicose veins
- skin care of stasis dermatitis

Actinic Keratosis

- topical 5-fluorouracil: dramatic response, but painful
- cryotherapy (liquid nitrogen) if only few lesions present

Malignant Melanoma

- prognosis depends on depth of invasion
- excisional biopsy (1-2 cm margins)
- if thin melanomas are completely excised patient can be considered "cured" but has a 10 fold higher risk of developing another melanoma
- if metastatic: radiotherapy and chemotherapy only of palliative value

Kaposi Sarcoma

- electrocoagulation for superficial lesions
- electron beam radiotherapy for deeper or unresponsive cases
- antineoplastic drugs in HIV positive patients will further reduce immunity !

MALIGNANCIES

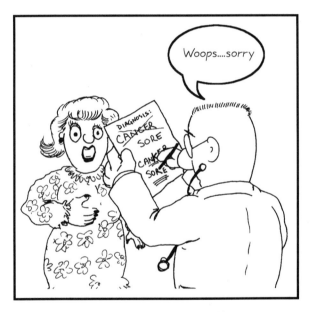

The hazards of poor spelling.

14.1.) <u>KEY-LIST</u>

14.2.) <u>TUMOR MARKERS</u>

occult blood	- positive if > 50 ml bleed - false negative: dietary vit. C - false positive: dietary meat, iron
PSA	**- prostate carcinoma** - more sensitive than acid phosphatase
CEA	**- adenocarcinomas** (colon, pancreas, lung) - non-neoplastic liver disease - Crohn's disease, ulcerative colitis
CA-125	**- ovarian cancer**
alpha-FP	**- hepatoma** - testicular tumor - neural tube defects - fetal death
alkaline phosphatase	**- obstructive biliary disease** **- bone metastases** - Paget's disease
acid phosphatase	- (benign prostatic hypertrophy) **- prostate carcinoma**

 None of these markers should be used for screening of otherwise asymptomatic patients (except possibly PSA).

14.3.) <u>PARANEOPLASTIC SYNDROMES</u>

DIC	- leukemias, lymphomas - adenocarcinomas
hypercalcemia	- squamous cell carcinoma (lung)
hypoglycemia	- insulinoma - mesenchymal tumors
thrombosis (Trousseau's syndrome)	- mucinous adenocarcinomas - myeloproliferative disorders
dermatomyositis	- breast and lung cancer
acanthosis nigricans	- stomach cancer
myasthenia (Lambert-Eaton)	- small cell carcinoma (lung)

14.4.) <u>PARAENDOCRINE SYNDROMES</u>

SIADH	- small cell carcinoma (lung)
Cushing's	- small cell carcinoma (lung)
flushing	- carcinoid
gynecomastia	- germ cell tumors - large cell carcinoma (lung)

GYNECOLOGY

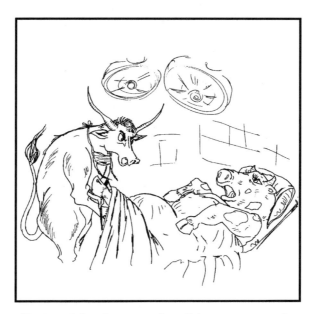

"Relax, Mrs. Benson. Don't have a cow."

15.1.) <u>SEX HORMONES</u>

hCG	**- pregnancy** urine: positive 3-4 weeks postconception serum RIA : positive on day 8 postconception - hydatidiform mole - choriocarcinoma
FSH	**- acts on granulosa cells** stimulates formation of LH receptors stimulates aromatization (testosterone -> estradiol)
LH	**- acts on theca cells** stimulates synthesis of testosterone **- acts on granulosa cells** transformation to corpus luteum
estrone	- principal estrogen of **menopause** - from peripheral conversion of androstenedione
estradiol	- more potent than estrone or estriol **- ovarian, testicular and adrenal tumors**
estriol	- mainly produced in **placenta**, but also requires fetus - used to monitor fetal well-being in high risk pregnancies

	FSH	LH
prepuberty	↓	↓
Stein-Leventhal	↓	↑
menopause	↑	↑

15.2.) <u>TANNER STAGES</u>

	male	female
1	- prepubertal - no pubic hair	- no breasts - no pubic hair
2	**- testicles enlarge** - scrotum reddens - some downy hair	**- breasts bud** - some downy hair
3	- some coarse, curly hair	**- enlargement of areolae** - breasts and areolae same level - some coarse, curly hair
4	- adult type hair (mons only)	**- areolae project above breasts** - adult type hair (mons only)
5	- hair spreads to medial thigh	- full breasts - hair spreads to medial thigh

 Menarche occurs at Tanner stage 3

 <u>***Peak of growth spurt***</u>*:*
Female : Tanner 2 (age 12)
Male   : Tanner 4 (age 14)

215

15.3.) <u>MENSTRUATION</u>

amenorrhea	- <u>primary</u>
	- absence of menses by **age 16**
	  if secondary sexual characteristics present
	- absence of menses by **age 14**
	  if secondary sexual characteristics absent
	
	- <u>secondary</u>
	- absence of menses more than 3 cycles

polymenorrhea	- intervals < 22 days
oligomenorrhea	- intervals > 40 days
hypomenorrhea	- regular bleeding, decreased amount
metrorrhagia	- irregular bleeding, normal amount
menorrhagia	- prolonged and excessive bleeding
DUB (dysfunctional uterine bleeding)	- excessive uterine bleeding - usually **anovulatory** (= estrogen breakthrough bleeding)

<u>Extra-info for the guys</u>:
- *normal is 30-50 ml over 4-5 days.*
- *anovulatory cycles (i.e. DUB) are normal for the first 1-2 years after menarche.*

15.4.) <u>PRIMARY AMENORRHEA</u>

Turner [1]	- XO
testicular feminization	- XY, testosterone receptor defect [2]
Müllerian dysgenesis	- absence of tubes, uterus, cervix, upper vagina
Stein-Leventhal (polycystic ovaries)	**- infertility, hirsutism**, endometrial hyperplasia **- high LH, androgens, estrogens** **- low or normal FSH**
Kallman syndrome	**- anosmia** - lack of GnRH
imperforate hymen	- monthly abdominal pain but no menses

[1] most common cause of primary amenorrhea

[2] testicles should be removed after full feminization is achieved !

15.5.) SECONDARY AMENORRHEA

stress, exercise	- leads to reduced GnRH levels
anorexia nervosa	- leads to reduced GnRH levels
post-pill	**- should last not longer than 6 months !**
drugs	- antipsychotics - tricyclic antidepressants - benzodiazepines - reserpine
Sheehan's	**- low FSH and LH**
pituitary neoplasms	**- increased prolactin**

 Pregnancy is the most common cause of secondary amenorrhea !

PROGESTERONE CHALLENGE TEST

positive if bleeding occurs.
- *patient is anovulatory*
  (no corpus luteum, no secretory transformation of endometrium)

negative if no bleeding within 2 weeks.
- *determine FSH levels*
- *CT scan of sella turcica*

15.6.) MENOPAUSE

- premature if age < 40 years

- follicles become less sensitive to gonadotropins
- **estrogen decreases**
- **LH and FSH increase** (up to 20 fold)

- vaginal bleeding due to unopposed estrogen normal for up to 12 months
- if vaginal bleeding continues > 12 months : rule out endometrial pathology

Estrogen replacement therapy :

advantages	disadvantages
Relief of menopausal symptoms - eliminates hot flashes - prevents atrophic vagina	**Absolute Contraindications** - liver disease - thrombosis, thrombophlebitis
Prevention of cardiovascular disease - decreases LDL - increases HDL	**Relative Contraindications** - hypertension - seizures
Prevention of osteoporosis - most effective if started early	**Increased cancer risk** - endometrial carcinoma: 4-8 fold - breast cancer: (controversial)

15.7.) <u>CONTRACEPTION</u>

	estimated pregnancy rate (during first year of "typical" use)
no method	85%
withdrawal method	25%
rhythm method	20%
diaphragm	20%
condom	15%
oral contraceptives	6%
IUD	4%
depot-progesterones (Norplant)	< 0.5%

Signs of ovulation : - *basal temperature increase by 0.5-1°F*
- *cervical mucus thin, watery, stretchy*
  ("Spinnbarkeit")

Contraindications for oral contraceptives *:*
- *pregnancy*
- *impaired liver function*
- *thrombophlebitis*
- *breast cancer, endometrial cancer*

15.8.) <u>INFERTILITY</u>

ovulatory factor	- abnormal androgen secretion - abnormal gonadotropin secretion - abnormal prolactin secretion
pelvic factor	- congenital abnormalities - salpingitis (gonorrhea, chlamydia) - endometriosis
cervical factor	- abnormal Pap smears - fetal DES exposure - mucos *(postcoital test)*
male factor	**- no sperm** - Klinefelter's - ductal obstruction - varicocele **- few sperm** - genetic - maturation arrest - heat **- abnormal morphology** - infections (mumps) **- abnormal motility** - infections (mumps) - immunologic incompatibility

***Overall causes*:**
50% women
30% men
20% combination of the two

15.9.) <u>NIPPLE DISCHARGE</u>

benign epithelial debris	- thick, grayish - common in middle-aged parous women
breast abscess	- thick, purulent
breast cancer	**- bloody or watery** - sometimes purulent
milky	- choriocarcinoma - drugs: phenothiazines 　　　　reserpine 　　　　cimetidine 　　　　oral contraceptives

 Most common cause of bloody nipple discharge:
benign intraductal papilloma !

15.10.) <u>BREAST CANCER</u>

fibrocystic disease	breast cancer
- often bilateral - multiple nodules - menstrual variation - may regress during pregnancy	- often unilateral - single mass - no cyclic variations

 Fibrocystic disease does not increase risk of breast cancer, but makes detection more difficult.

perhaps benign	perhaps malignant
- discrete, smooth - movable - tender	- ill-defined, thickened - non-movable - edema
<u>mammogram</u> - round, ovoid, smooth - clearly defined margins - may contain calcifications	<u>mammogram</u> - distinct, irregular tumor mass - projection of dense spicules - may contain calcifications

> *<u>risk factors</u>:*
> *- family history*
> *- age of patient*
> *- (estrogens)*

15.11.) <u>OVARIAN CANCER</u>

Most common presentation: vague abdominal complaints.

Stage I	- confined to 1 or 2 ovaries
Stage II	- pelvic spread
Stage III	- intraabdominal spread
Stage IV	- distant spread

> ### *risk factors:*
> - *low parity*
> - *history of miscarriages or infertility*
> - *subclinical mumps*
> - *breast cancer*
> - *diet rich in animal fats*

15.12.) <u>ENDOMETRIAL CANCER</u>

 Most common presentation: abnormal uterine bleeding.

Stage I	- limited to **endometrium**
Stage II	- involves **endocervical glands or stroma**
Stage III	- invades **serosa** - or involves **vagina** - or pelvic and/or paraaortic lymph nodes
Stage IV	- involves **rectum or bladder** - or distant metastases

---

***risk factors*:**
- *obesity*
- *nulliparity*
- *estrogen use*
- *pelvic radiation*

15.13.) <u>VAGINAL DISCHARGE</u>

Candida	- white, curd-like - sweet odor
Chlamydia	- yellow, mucopurulent - odorless
Trichomonas	- frothy, greenish - foul smelling
Gardnerella	- green/gray - foul smelling - **clue cells**: epithelial cells with cocci - **whiff test**: add KOH to discharge -> fishy smell
Gonorrhea	- in 80%: asymptomatic - in 20%: yellowish green discharge from Bartholini's glands

15.14.) <u>CERVICITIS / STDS</u>

	signs & symptoms	diagnosis
chlamydia	- often asymptomatic - or cervicitis	- culture
gonorrhea [1]	- asymptomatic - or purulent discharge	- culture (Thayer-Martin)
syphilis	- chancre sore - fever - skin rash (secondary)	- VDRL - FTAbs
herpes	- multiple tender vesicles - fever (if primary)	
chancroid	soft, painful ulcer	- biopsy
human papilloma virus	- warts - painless	

---

[1]*<u>Pelvic Inflammatory Disease</u>:*
   1. cervicitis (50% asymptomatic)
   2. salpingitis (often also few symptoms)
   3. peritoneal adhesions (uterus, adnexae)
      dyspareunia, sterility, chronic aching pelvic pain

15.15.) CERVICAL CANCER - 1

Pap smear (Bethesda Classification) :

benign cellular changes	**infection** - Trichomonas infection - Candida infection **reactive changes** - inflammation - atrophic vaginitis
epithelial cell abnormalities	**atypical squamous cells of undetermined significance** (borderline between severe reactive change and mild dysplasia) **lowgrade intraepithelial lesion** - human papilloma virus - mild dysplasia (CIN 1) **highgrade intraepithelial lesion** - moderate dysplasia (CIN 2) - severe dysplasia (CIN 3) - carcinoma in situ **Squamous cell carcinoma**

False negative rate of Pap smear: 15 - 35%

Highgrade lesions are more likely to progress to invasive carcinoma than lowgrade lesions, but the biological potential in any individual patient is uncertain.

228

15.16.) <u>CERVICAL CANCER - 2</u>

Stage I	- carcinoma **limited to cervix**
Stage II	- involvement of **upper 2/3 vagina** - or involvement of parametria
Stage III	- involvement of **lower 1/3 vagina** - or involvement of **pelvic sidewall**
Stage IV	- involvement of **bladder or rectum** - or distant metastases

---

<u>risk factors</u>:
- *multiple sex partners at early age*
- *human papilloma virus (especially types 16 and 18)*
- *smoking*

Hot-List

Primary Amenorrhea
- if uterus absent: karyotype
- if uterus present and vagina patent: workup like secondary amenorrhea

Secondary Amenorrhea
- if hirsutism present: rule out polycystic ovaries, ovarian and adrenal tumors
- progestin challenge and FSH to distinguish between hypothalamic and gonadal failure
- prolactinoma: transsphenoidal destruction of pituitary adenoma. Induce ovulation with bromocriptine

Dysmenorrhea
- NSAIDs (ibuprofen)
- oral contraceptives -> anovulation -> decreased prostaglandin production
- adenomyosis and endometriosis may require surgical treatment

Polycystic Ovary
- weight loss
- clomiphene to induce ovulation
- ovarian wedge resection rarely necessary
- endometrial biopsies to exclude cancer

Infertility
- **male factor**: semen analysis, postcoital test, consider removal of varicocele, consider sperm aspiration and IVF
- **ovarian factor**: document ovulation (basal temperature, progesterone levels), induce with clomiphene, bromocriptine for anovulation due to prolactin excess.
- **cervical factor**: treat chronic infections, mucus quality, test behavior of sperms in mucus, consider steroids if antisperm antibodies present
- **tubal factor**: determine patency, IVF
- **uterine factor**: treat endometritis, consider removal of myomas

Toxic Shock Syndrome

- aggressive supportive therapy: Fluid and electrolytes, antibiotics
- monitor urine output and pulmonary wedge pressure
- consider replacement of coagulation factors
- Causes of death: 1. respiratory distress syndrome 2. cardiovascular failure 3. hemorrhage (DIC)

Endometriosis

- **induce "pseudopregnancy":** maintain high progesterone levels (side-effects: depression, constipation, weight gain, breakthrough bleeding)
- **induce "pseudomenopause":** reduce estrogen and progesterone levels
  - danazol (weak androgen) suppresses gonadotropin release
  - GnRH agonists

Pelvic Inflammatory Disease

- empirical antibiotic treatment (e.g. ceftriaxone plus doxycycline)
- hospitalize if temperature >102.2 °F or signs of peritonitis (guarding, rebound tenderness) are present
- examine and treat all male partners

Bartholin's Gland Abscess

- drainage (Ward catheter). Simple incision and drainage provides temporary relief only

Fibrocystic Disease

- FNA: clear fluid: observe. Residual mass or bloody: excisional biopsy
- avoid trauma
- giving up coffee and tea may help

Fibroadenoma

- excision under local anesthesia

Breast Cancer

- lumpectomy (most popular for early stages)
- simple mastectomy: breast removal, lymph nodes left in place
- modified radical mastectomy: removal of breast, pectoralis major fascia (but not muscle) and lymph nodes
- radical mastectomy: en-bloc removal of breast, pectoral muscles and axillary nodes
- adjuvant chemotherapy if axillary nodes positive
- tamoxifen if estrogen receptor positive

Ovarian Cancer

- surgical removal plus chemotherapy
- dysgerminomas: chemotherapy or radiotherapy

Uterine Leiomyoma

- if asymptomatic or patient postmenopause: no treatment necessary
- consider removal if excessively large (>12weeks uterus)

Endometrial Cancer

- hysterectomy plus radiation therapy
- progesterone
- chemotherapy for metastases (doxorubicin, cisplatin)

Cervical Cancer

- Pap-smear: If Class II or above -> colposcopy and biopsy
- If biopsy shows microinvasion (Stage IA) -> cone biopsy

OBSTETRICS

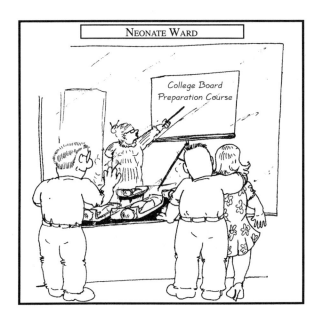

16.1.) <u>DRUGS DURING PREGNANCY</u>

	safe	unsafe
hypertension	β-blockers	thiazides ACE inhibitors
diabetes	insulin	sulfonylureas
asthma	cromolyn terbutaline	steroids
analgesics	acetaminophen	ibuprofen indomethacin
antibiotics	penicillins sulfonamides erythromycin amphotericin B	quinine tetracyclines
anticoagulants	heparin	warfarin

<u>*Some common drugs to avoid*</u>
<u>*during breast feeding:*</u>
- *antineoplastic agents*
- *bromocriptine*
- *cimetidine*
- *ergotamines*
- *gold salts*
- *lithium*
- *thiouracil*

 Do not breast feed with HIV, chronic HBV or CMV infection !

16.2.) <u>PARITY</u>

nulligravida	- is not and never has been pregnant
primigravida	- is or has been pregnant - irrespective of pregnancy outcome
nullipara	- has never completed a pregnancy - may or may not have aborted
primipara	- has completed one pregnancy (> 500g , dead or alive)
multipara	- has completed two or more pregnancies

 A women with her first triplets is also primipara !

235

16.3.) <u>PREGNANCY SIGNS</u>

presumptive signs	**menses** > 10 days late
	morning nausea - occurs at 4-6 weeks of gestation
	breast changes - tenderness - enlargement of Montgomery's tubercles
	chloasma - darkening of skin over forehead, bridge of nose and cheekbones
	quickening - first perception of fetal movement - occurs at 16-20 weeks

probable signs	**uterus enlarged**
	  12 weeks : above symphysis
	  20 weeks : at umbilicus

	Hegar's sign softening of cervix
	Chadwick's sign bluish discoloration of cervix
	hCG or β-hCG
certain signs	**fetal heart tones** 17-19 weeks by auscultation
	ultrasound identification after 6 weeks

 Nägele's rule : *9 month plus 7 days from beginning of LMP.*

16.4.) PREGNANCY SCREENS

initial	- hemoglobin - blood group, Rh factor - rubella titers - syphilis (VDRL) - Pap smear - if at risk: HBV, HIV, toxoplasmosis

urine test	- *if bacteriuria (> 10^5/ml): treat !*
	  (even if asymptomatic)
	
	- glucosuria is common !
	  (not important if blood sugar is normal)

at 16 weeks	**triple screen (for Down's)** - AFP, hCG, estriol - *if abnormal : amniocentesis*
amniocentesis	- offer to women > 35 years - previous chromosomal abnormality - history of spontaneous abortions - usually done between **16-18th week** - < 1% risk of fetal loss
chorionic villi sample	- best done between **9th-11th week** - 5% risk of fetal loss

AFP elevated:	- *open neural tube* - *multiple gestation* - *duodenal atresia*
AFP decreased:	- *Down syndrome*

16.5.) <u>PREGNANCY BLEEDING</u>

first trimester	- **very common** - 50% result in spontaneous abortion - 50% continue as normal pregnancy
second trimester	- low lying placenta

third trimester	- **bloody show** : mixed with mucos, labor
	
	- **placentia previa : heavy, painless bleeding** [1]
	
	- **abruptio placentae : none or heavy bleeding**
	                    continuous abdominal pain
	                    sustained uterine contraction
	                    fetal distress
	                    DIC
	
	- **uterus rupture** : sudden cessation of uterine contractions
	                    disappearance of fetal heart tones

puerperium	- normal up to 500 ml blood loss - hypotonic uterus [2] - ruptured uterus - retention of placental tissue - trauma (lacerations, episiotomy)

[1] do not palpate cervix unless ready for delivery !
[2] common if general anesthesia is used (try massage of uterus or oxytocin).

 Kleihauer-Betke test:
fetal RBCs are more resistant to alkaline pH than maternal RBCs.

16.6.) PREGNANCY COMPLICATIONS

gestational diabetes	- glucosuria commonly due to increased GFR
	- glucola: 1h oral glucose tolerance test
	
	- **risks** : preeclampsia
	        infections
	        large infants
	        neural tube defects
	
	- *diet or insulin*

hypertension	- 140/90 or more than 30 mmHg systolic rise - in early pregnancy : suggests mole - *hospitalization, bed rest*
preeclampsia	- hypertension plus proteinuria - more common in nullipara - *hydralazine, Mg^{2+}-sulfate (anticonvulsive)* - *delivery*
eclampsia	- preeclampsia plus convulsions
heart disease (see 4.14)	**class I, II** - can go through pregnancy **class III** - may be indication for abortion - deliver vaginal ! - **class IV** - high mortality (cardiac failure)

239

16.7.) <u>SPONTANEOUS ABORTION</u>

threatened abortion	- bleeding - uterine cramping **- no cervical dilation**
inevitable abortion	- bleeding - uterine cramping **- ruptured membranes** **- cervix dilated**
incomplete abortion	**- retained placental tissue**
early abortion	- very common (~50% of all conceptions) - often unnoticed - usually due to chromosomal abnormalities
missed abortion	**- death of fetus or embryo** - no labor or passage of tissue
habitual abortion	- three or more spontaneous abortions

> ***Causes of habitual abortion*:**
> - *defective zygote*
> - *cervical incompetence*
> - *infections*
> - *hormonal dysfunction*
> - *chromosomal abnormalities*

16.8.) <u>LABOR</u>

	true labor	false labor
intervals	regular	irregular
contraction	intensity increases gradually	intensity constant
sedation	does not affect contractions	stops contractions

first stage	- about 12 hours (primipara) - cervix effacement and dilation - **latent phase** : slow dilation of cervix - **active phase** : dilation > 1.2 cm/h
second stage	- about 1 hour (primipara) - delivery of infant
third stage	- within 5 min. - delivery of placenta

 Indications for induction of labor :
- ruptured membranes > 48h
- chorioamnionitis

<u>**Stations are measured in cm below level of ischial spine:**</u>
O station   = engagement
+1 station   = presenting part 1 cm below ischial spine
+2 station   = presenting part 2 cm below ischial spine
               ⋮

16.9.) <u>LABOR PATTERNS</u>

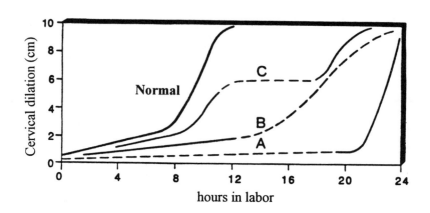

From *Obstetrics and Gynecology*, 2nd edition, p. 190, by C.R.B. Beckmann et al.
Copyright 1995 by Williams & Wilkins, Baltimore, MD. Used with permission.

A: prolonged latent phase
B: prolonged active phase
C: arrest of active phase

<u>PREMATURE RUPTURE OF MEMBRANES</u>

- danger of chorioamnionitis
- amniotic fluid shows ferning
- amniotic fluid has pH > 7.0 (Nitrazine test)

- **amniotic band syndrome**: - fetus becomes entangled in membranes
  - resulting in deformities, finger amputations...

16.10.) <u>PREMATURITY</u>

- gestational age **20-28 weeks : immature**
- gestational age **28-37 weeks : premature**
  (irrespective of birth weight or fetal maturity)

> risk factors : - African-Americans
> - low socioeconomic status
> - previous premature births
> - **smoking**

- *monitor risk patients : weekly cervical exams*

- **cervical incompetence** : history of second trimester abortions in
  absence of uterine contractions

- **L/S ratio** preferably > 2

16.11.) <u>POSTMATURITY</u>

- gestational age **42 weeks or more**
  irrespective of birth weight or fetal maturity

- signs of dysmaturity : dry, wrinkled skin, loss of subcutaneous fat,
  meconium staining, long nails

nonstress test	- 3 or more fetal movements in 30 min - heart rate accelerations > 15 beats/min
oxytocin stress test	- **negative**: no or early deceleration - **positive**: late decelerations
biophysical profile (ultrasound)	1. nonstress test 2. fetal breathing, 3. tone and 4. motion 5. amount of amniotic fluid

243

16.12.) <u>THE FETUS</u>

fetal lie	**- long axis of fetus in relation to long axis of uterus** - longitudinal - transverse - oblique

fetal presentation	**- portion of fetus that can be felt through cervix**
	
	- **cephalic** : vertex
	               face
	               brow
	
	- **frank breech** (thighs are flexed, legs are extended)
	
	- **complete breech** (thighs are flexed, legs are flexed)
	
	- footling breech

fetal position	**- relation of fetal occiput[1] to maternal birth canal** - left occiput anterior - left occiput transverse - left occiput posterior etc....

[1] or chin in case of face presentation.

16.13.) <u>FETAL HEART RATE</u>

normal	- **good variability** (120 to 160 beats/min)
absent variability	- high perinatal mortality !
early decelerations	- not a/w poor fetal outcome - not caused by hypoxemia
late decelerations	- **fetal hypoxemia** - myocardial compression - a/w hypertension, preeclampsia, maternal hypotension, excessive uterine contractions (oxytocin)
variable decelerations	- transient compression of umbilical cord

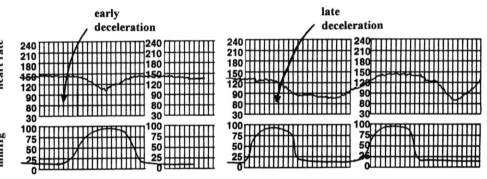

From *Obstetrics and Gynecology*, 2nd edition, p. 201, by C.R.B. Beckmann et al.
Copyright 1995 by Williams & Wilkins, Baltimore, MD. Used with permission.

Management of late decelerations:
 - *if late decelerations persist sample fetal scalp blood and monitor pH.*
 - *if pH < 7.25 repeat every 30 min.*
 - *if pH < 7.20 deliver !*

16.14.) ANESTHESIA

paracervical block	**- relieves pain from uterine contractions** - not sufficient for labor - may cause fetal bradycardia
pudendal block	**- for spontaneous delivery** - for repair of episiotomy - not sufficient for forceps delivery - may cause systemic toxicity
epidural anesthesia	**- for vaginal delivery or c-section** - not always effective analgesia (not enough for perineum) - inadvertent subarachnoid blockade may cause systemic and CNS toxicity
spinal anesthesia (subarachnoid)	**- for vaginal delivery or c-section** - <u>compared to epidural</u>: - more rapid onset - less fetal toxicity - higher risk of severe maternal hypotension
general anesthesia	- for emergencies or if spinal/epidural are contraindicated - **NO_2** : - does not interfere with uterine contractions - does not prolong labor - **halothane** : may cause atonic uterus -> hemorrhage

 If hemorrhage or coagulation disorders are present, spinal and epidural anesthesia are contraindicated.

16.15.) <u>EPISIOTOMY</u>

	midline	mediolateral
advantages	- easy to repair - small blood loss - minimal post-op. pain - rare dyspareunia	- more space for breech deliveries
disadvantages	- **may extend** (into anal sphincter)	- **more difficult to repair** - greater blood loss - commonly post-op. pain - dyspareunia

16.16.) <u>TROPHOBLASTIC DISEASE</u>

hydatidiform mole	choriocarcinoma
- diffuse hydropic chorionic villi - hyperplastic trophoblasts	- proliferation of cytotrophoblast - proliferation of syncytiotrophoblast - no villi present
- vaginal bleeding - uterine size greater than date - hyperemesis	**- following molar pregnancy** **- following spontaneous abortion** **- following term pregnancy**
- high β-hCG	- high β-hCG
- invasive mole : invades myometrium	

<u>*complete mole:*</u>
- *empty oocyte fertilized by sperm*
- *46XX (both X are paternal origin)*

<u>*incomplete mole:*</u>
- *mole plus fetal remnants*
- *triploid set of chromosomes*

Hot-List

Hyperemesis
- small frequent meals (light and dry)
- high dose vit. B6 may help
- use antinausea drugs only as last resort
- hospitalize if patient is dehydrated and ketonuric

Gestational Diabetes
- glucosuria is unreliable finding
- glucola (50g sugar) screening test
- diet and exercise
- close monitoring of blood glucose and fetal growth
- glucose tolerance should return to normal postpartum, but 50% risk to develop diabetes mellitus in the future

Preeclampsia
- hospitalize !
- monitor proteinuria
- monitor fetus. Corticosteroids to accelerate lung maturation
- past 28 weeks, if preeclampsia is severe: deliver !
- anticonvulsants (Mg^{2+} sulfate) during labor !

Eclampsia
- seizures: Mg^{2+} sulfate or phenytoin
- hypertension: hydralazine or labetalol
- attempt labor. If eclampsia severe: cesarean section

Ectopic Pregnancy
- culdocentesis: non-clotting blood indicates bleeding from ruptured ectopic gestation
- exploratory laparoscopy . If bleeding is profound: laparotomy

Abruptio Placentae
- if concealed, bleeding is not apparent (worst prognosis)
- rupture membranes and prepare delivery
- if fetus is dead or questionable: vaginal delivery
  if placenta separation is limited and fetus monitored: vaginal delivery
- if hemorrhage uncontrollable (maternal indication): c-section
  if fetus viable but under distress (fetal indication): c-section

Placenta Previa
- avoid vaginal examination
- confirm or rule out by ultrasound
- cesarean section

Premature Rupture of Membranes
- if gestational age > 33 weeks: deliver to reduce risk of amnionitis
- if gestational age < 33 weeks: determine fetal lung maturity. Give corticosteroids to accelerate maturation. Closely monitor patient for signs of infection
- if gestational age <26 weeks: little hope for fetal survival

Premature Labor
- emergency: tocolytic agents (terbutaline), $MgSO_4$
- continued care: oral β-sympathomimetics

Incompetent Cervix
- rule out preterm labor !
- prophylactic cerclage may be placed at 12-16 weeks

Prolonged Labor
- exclude fetopelvic disproportion
- supportive measures
- avoid excessive sedation or regional anesthesia
- avoid oxytocin if contractions are already adequate

Postpartum Hemorrhage

- uterine atony: try massage first. If it doesn't work: Methylergonovine, oxytocin or PGF2α
- rule out uterus inversion (requires immediate manual replacement)

Postpartum Sepsis

- if temperature > 100.4 °F within first 24h after delivery
- Chlamydia, Bacteroides, Mycoplasma
- bed rest (semi-Fowler position), antibiotics

Postpartum Depression

- occurs most commonly between day 3 and 10 postpartum

Postpartum Thrombophlebitis

- early ambulation
- consider prophylaxis for phlebothrombosis
- advise not to use oral contraceptives
- advise to stop smoking

Hydatidiform Mole

- dilation and suction
- sharp curettage
- hysterectomy not necessary
- monitor β-hCG for 6-12 months

Choriocarcinoma

- chemotherapy
- cure rate almost 100%
- future pregnancies possible

PEDIATRICS

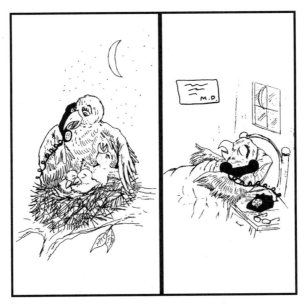

**"Just keep feeding them on demand, Mrs. Rogers.
Some children need more than others."**

17.1.) <u>BIRTH TRAUMA - 1</u>

periventr. hemorrhage **intraventr. hemorrhage**	**- often occurs without obvious trauma** - vulnerability to cerebral blood flow and pressure changes - in small or preterm infants - hypotension, bradycardia, apnea - lethargy, seizures, coma
subdural hemorrhage	**- mechanical trauma, forceps** (cephalopelvic disproportion) - more common in large infants
cephalhematoma	- subperiostal hemorrhage **- limited to area of affected bone**
caput succedaneum	- diffuse edema of scalp soft tissue **- not limited to area of bones**

17.2.) <u>BIRTH TRAUMA - 2</u>

clavicle fracture	- usually "green-stick" - initially often asymptomatic
Erb-Duchenne	- **injury of superior brachial plexus (C5, C6)** - due to lateral pull of head during shoulder extraction - **"waiter's tip" position** (forearm extended and internally rotated, wrist flexed) - absent biceps reflex
Klumpke	- **injury of inferior brachial plexus (C8, T1)** - (distal paralysis) wrist drop - Horner's syndrome common
amnion band syndrome	- a/w early rupture of membranes - loss of a digit or limb due to constriction

17.3.) __APGAR SCORE__

	0	**1**	**2**
heart rate	none	< 100/min	> 100/min
respiratory effort	none	slow, irregular	good, crying
muscle tone	limp	some flexion	active motion
reflex irritability	absent	grimace	cough or sneeze
color	blue, pale	acrocyanosis	pink

reproduced with permission from : Apgar et al., JAMA 168:1985-88, 1958

 - 7 or above is good.
 - Apgar score does not indicate long term prognosis.

17.4.) <u>SUBSTANCE ABUSE DURING PREGNANCY</u>

heroin, PCP	- no congenital abnormalities **neonatal withdrawal** - jitteriness - hyperreflexia - seizures
cocaine	- placenta abruption ! - increased risk for SIDS
inhalants	- neurotoxicity - microcephaly
tobacco	- increased frequency of abortion - low birth weight

 Testing maternal urine for drugs requires consent !
Testing infant's blood or urine for drugs does not require consent !

17.5.) <u>TERATOGENS</u>

alcohol	**- microphthalmia** **- short palpebral fissures** - flat nasal bridge - broad upper lip
retinoids	**- severe CNS abnormalities** - congenital heart defects - ear malformations (small or absent)
diphenylhydantoin	**- hypoplasia of distal phalanges** **- small nails** - flat nasal bridge - cleft lip/palate
warfarin	**- chondrodysplasia** (stippled vertebral and femoral epiphyses) - nasal hypoplasia
thalidomide	- upper limb phocomelia - lower limb phocomelia

Retinoic acid cream (for treatment of acne) should also be avoided during pregnancy, even though its systemic concentration is too low to be teratogenic.

17.6.) <u>CONGENITAL INFECTIONS</u>

toxoplasmosis	**T** **O**	- hydrocephalus - **generalized calcifications** - chorioretinitis
rubella	**R**	- heart defects - microcephaly, microphthalmia - **cataracts** - **hearing loss**
CMV	**C**	- microcephaly, microphthalmia - **periventricular calcifications** - chorioretinitis
herpes	**H**	- microphthalmia - retinopathy - intracranial calcifications
syphilis		**newborns often asymptomatic** **3-12 weeks:** - jaundice - hemolytic anemia - rhinitis ("snuffles") - rash on palms and soles **permanent stigma:** - Hutchinson's teeth - saddle nose - saber shins
varicella		- **limb hypoplasia** - cutaneous scars - cortical atrophy

17.7.) __TRISOMIES__

	features	life expectancy	prenatal survival	recurrence risk
trisomy 21	- congenital heart defects - mongoloid eye slant - depressed nasal bridge - protruding tongue - transverse palmar crease	50% live > 50 years (early Alzheimer's)	25% [1]	about 1% [2]
trisomy 18	- clenched hands - overlapping 2nd and 5th finger - low set ears - short sternum - nail hypoplasia	90% die in first month	5%	< 1%
trisomy 13	- severe CNS abnormalities - microphthalmia - polydactyly - cleft lip / palate	100% lethal by 6 months	1%	< 1%

[1] i.e. 75% are spontaneously aborted.
[2] recurrence risk is higher if due to translocation !

17.8.) <u>MULTIFACTORIAL BIRTH DEFECTS</u>

cleft lip / cleft palate	- cleft lip (with or without cleft palate) is genetically distinct form isolated cleft palate.
anencephaly **spina bifida**	- a/w folate deficiency.
congenital heart defects	- common component of many syndromes.

17.9.) PERINATAL VIRAL INFECTIONS

varicella	**- if mother infected within days of delivery** - maybe severe, disseminated - often fatal encephalitis *- give immunoglobulin after birth*
herpes simplex	**- high risk if primary maternal infection** - low risk if recurrent maternal infection - herpetic encephalitis *- c-section if active lesions present*
hepatitis B	- usually results in chronic subclinical hepatitis - rarely fulminant hepatitis *- screen all pregnant women for HBsAg* *- c-section not necessary* *- give immunoglobulin after birth*
HIV [1]	**typical onset of symptoms 4-6 months after birth** - lymphadenopathy - hepatomegaly - splenomegaly - failure to thrive *- c-section not helpful (transplacental transfer !)* *- AZT*

[1] IgG antibodies in < 9 month old infant may be of maternal origin !

perinatal infections	:	*infection near term.*
congenital syndromes	:	*infection in early pregnancy causing specific birth defects.*

17.10.) <u>RESPIRATORY DISTRESS SYNDROME</u>
(hyaline membrane disease)

risk factors	- male sex - premature birth - second born twin - perinatal asphyxia - maternal diabetes - L/S ratio < 2
clinical features	- tachypnea - nasal flaring - grunting - cyanosis - "ground glass" appearance on CXR
complications	**intrinsic:** - pneumothorax - pulmonary emphysema **oxygen therapy:** - bronchopulmonary dysplasia - retinopathy

17.11.) <u>MECONIUM ASPIRATION SYNDROME</u>

risk factors	- some meconium staining of amniotic fluid is seen in up to 15% of normal pregnancies - meconium is passed during intrauterine stress - more common in post term infants
clinical features	- cyanosis, tachypnea - persistent pulmonary hypertension

17.12.) <u>NEONATAL CONJUNCTIVITIS</u>

chemical	**- within first 2 days after birth** - due to silver nitrate
gonorrheal	**- 1 to 2 weeks after birth** - prevent with silver nitrate or erythromycin
chlamydial	**- 1 to 2 weeks after birth** - watch for systemic infection (i.e. pneumonia)
viral	- most common cause in **infants > 3 months** - usually adenovirus

<u>*Symptoms*</u> :
- *purulent discharge*
- *eye lid reddening or swelling*

- *Mucous drainage from eye for 1-2 days after birth is normal and*
  does not indicate conjunctivitis !

 Constant tearing after birth indicates blockage of
nasolacrimal duct.

17.13.) <u>NEONATAL HYPERBILIRUBINEMIA</u>

	UC	C	
physiologic jaundice	X		- **3 to 5 days postnatal** - due to increased bilirubin production and relatively immature liver
breast milk jaundice	X		- **2 to 3 weeks after birth** - due to increased bilirubin absorption - *brief interruption of breast feeding* *(usually not necessary)*
hemolysis	X		- Rh, ABO incompatibility - spherocytosis - G6PDH deficiency

enzyme defects	X		- **Gilbert** (mild)
			  (decreased hepatic bilirubin uptake)
			
			- **Crigler-Naijar** (severe)
			  (deficient glucuronyl transferase)

		X	- **Dubin Johnson** (impaired hepatocellular secretion)
cholestasis		X	- bile duct stenosis - biliary atresia - hepatitis - cystic fibrosis
kernicterus	X		- **unconjugated bilirubin > 20 mg/dl** - staining of basal ganglia - lethargy, hypotonia, encephalopathy

UC : mainly unconjugated bilirubin   **C** : mainly conjugated bilirubin

17.14.) <u>SMALL & LARGE INFANTS</u>

SGA	LGA
2 SD below expected	**2 SD above expected**
- chromosomal abnormalities - TORCH - alcohol, drug abuse - maternal hypertension - placenta insufficiency	- diabetic mother - genetic/ racial - Prader Willi

Low birthweight infant : *< 2500 g at birth*
(can be SGA, AGA or LGA)

<u>Problems of infants of diabetic mothers</u>:
 - birth trauma
- hypoglycemia
- respiratory distress syndrome

- L/S ratio is <u>not reliable</u> for infants of diabetic mothers !
- better: amniotic fluid phosphatidyl glycerin.

17.15.) NUTRITION

breast milk [1]	**compared to cow milk:** - more fat - more carbohydrates - more lactalbumin, less casein - both lack vit. D !
supplementation	**iron** - start supplementation at age **4-6 months** (earlier in preterm infants) **fluoride** - for all breast fed infants - or if Fl⁻ content of drinking water is poor Ca^{2+} , **vit. D** - for breast fed infants at risk (little sunlight etc.) **vit. B12** - for breast fed infants if mother is vegetarian
commercial formulas	**cow milk based** (with added whey protein) **soy protein formulas** - "hypoallergenic", but cross-reactivity is common - useful after diarrhea (transient lactase deficiency)

[1] *10% weight loss by 2 weeks is normal for breast fed infants.*

 Human milk is best for humans, cow milk is best for calves.

Viruses that can be transmitted via breast milk:
- hepatitis B *- HIV* *- rubella* *- herpes* *- CMV*

17.16.) <u>GROWTH CURVES</u>

**Height
or
Weight**

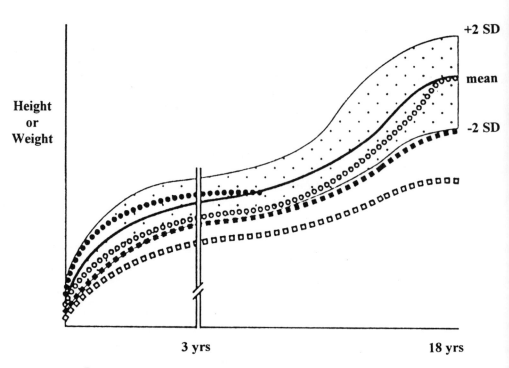

+2 SD

mean

-2 SD

3 yrs

18 yrs

From *Rudolph's Pediatrics*, 20th edition, page 4, edited by A.M. Rudolph.
Copyright 1996 by Appleton & Lange. Used with permission.

Postnatal-onset pathologic growth	●
Constitutional growth delay	○
Genetic short stature	■
Prenatal-onset pathologic growth	□

268

17.17.) <u>INFECTIOUS DISEASES OF CHILDHOOD - 1</u>

rubeola (measles)	- 8 to 12 days incubation
	- **3 to 5 days prodromal**
	  (cough, coryza, conjunctivitis)
	
	- followed by Koplik's spots
	- then maculopapular rash
	  neck -> face -> arms -> trunk
	
	- subacute sclerosing panencephalitis
	  (rare but deadly)

rubella (German measles)	- 14 to 21 days incubation
	- **mild prodrome, tender lymph nodes**
	
	- maculopapular rash, 3 day fever
	  neck -> face -> arms -> trunk
	
	- infection during first trimester results in
	  30% chance of congenital abnormalities

roseola (exanthema subitum)	- acute high fever - **maculopapular rash as fever falls** - rash begins on trunk

17.18.) <u>INFECTIOUS DISEASES OF CHILDHOOD - 2</u>

varicella (chickenpox)	- 11 to 21 days incubation - mild prodrome, anorexia **- generalized pruritic vesicles** - begin on trunk -> face, extremities - lesions at different stages of healing *- patients with herpes zoster can transmit* *virus to susceptible children !*
fifth disease **(erythema infectiosum)**	- 7 days incubation - no prodrome, no fever - sudden bright rash **"slapped cheeks"** then maculopapular rash on trunk and extremities - complication: aplastic anemia
scarlet fever	- 1 to 7 days incubation - pharyngitis - rapid onset fever, headache, vomiting **- "sand paper" rash** **- starts at time of fever** **- spares the face** - strawberry tongue

17.19.) <u>RESPIRATORY TRACT INFECTIONS</u>

croup	- usually viral - **gradual onset** - low fever - stridor improves with epinephrine	**parainfluenza**
epiglottitis [1]	- **acute onset** - high fever - some relief with neck extension ("sniffing dog position") - "thumb-print sign" on x-ray	**hemophilus influenzae**
tracheitis	- **gradual onset** - high fever - subglottal narrowing	bacterial (**Staph. aureus**)
bronchiolitis	- children 2 to 6 months - variable fever - respiratory distress - rhonchi, wheezes, rales - does not respond to bronchodilators	viral (**RSV**)

 [1] *do not examine with tongue blade unless ready to intubate !*

17.20.) <u>RHEUMATIC FEVER</u>

major criteria	- **carditis** - **polyarthritis** - **chorea** - **erythema marginatum** - **subcutaneous nodules**
minor criteria	- fever - arthralgia - elevated acute phase reactants

- ***ASO titer*** *performed to confirm <u>past</u> infection with Group A β-hemolytic streptococci*

- ***rapid antigen assay*** *if suspected acute infection.*
- *if negative result and still suspected: throat swab and culture.*

- *Penicillin within 10 days of infection prevents rheumatic fever.*

17.21.) CHILDHOOD TUMORS

Wilms' tumor	- **typical age : 2-5 years** - **typical presentation : asymptomatic abdominal mass** - arises anywhere within kidney (*distorts* urinary collecting system) - survival about 85%

neuroblastoma	- **typical age : 2 years**
	- **typical presentation : asymptomatic abdominal mass**
	- arises from neural crest
	   (*displaces* urinary collecting system)
	- survival about 80% in young children
	   (poorer in older children)

Ewing's sarcoma	- **typical age : 10-15 years** - **severe limb pain (causing awakening at night)** - arises from medullary cavity (commonly : femur) - survival < 40%
histiocytosis [1]	- **typical age : infants, young children** - **typical presentation: fever, weight loss, anemia** - multiple disease entities - lytic bone lesions - may resolve spontaneously or require chemotherapy
brain tumors	- infratentorial more common than supratentorial - astrocytoma more common than medulloblastoma - MRI is study of choice - no lumbar puncture (risk of herniation !)

[1] *Langerhans cells are normal phagocytic skin cells.*

17.22.) <u>CHILD ABUSE</u>

perhaps accidental	perhaps intentional
- splash marks - injuries to front - foot soles spared	- clearly demarcated areas, no splash - injuries to back - foot soles involved - history of multiple injuries - retinal hemorrhage (shaken baby)

 *As physician **you are not supposed to play detective.** If you suspect abuse, report it to the Department of Social Services.*

> ***Forms of abuse**:*
> *- physical*
> *- emotional*
> *- sexual*
> *- neglect*

Hot-List

INFECTIONS / IMMUNOLOGY

AIDS
- HIV antibody test unreliable in children < 15 months
- vaccinate at usual intervals, but give inactivated polio rather than oral
- AZT, aggressive treatment of infections

Meningitis
- lumbar puncture and blood culture if any suspicion
- empiric treatment: ampicillin plus cefotaxime
- if seizures develop: suspect encephalitis

Measles
- supportive only
- avoid salicylates (better: acetaminophen)
- immunoglobulin effective if given within first 6 days

Rubella
- teratogenic (especially during first trimester)
- seropositive mothers are immune
- seroconversion in first trimester indicates high risk (consider abortion)

Mumps
- supportive only
- orchitis: analgesics and scrotal support
- unilateral nerve deafness: usually transient

Chicken Pox

- supportive measures, trim nails
- diphenhydramine for itching
- prevent secondary bacterial infections
- acyclovir (topical or systemic) for ocular infection

Pertussis

- Erythromycin for patient and household contacts (regardless of age or immunization status)
- nutritional support
- cough suppressants of little benefit

Henoch Schönlein Purpura

- usually self limited: supportive care only
- corticosteroids if gastrointestinal hemorrhage present

CONGENITAL HEART DISEASE

ASD

- determine pulmonary vs. systemic blood flow (cardiac catheter oximetry)
- if > 2:1 consider surgical correction (best done at ages 2-4 years)
- if untreated: shunt reversal and heart failure common in third and fourth decade.

VSD

- if small expect spontaneous closure
- elective surgery at 2-4 years
- significant pulmonary hypertension is a contraindication for surgery !

PDA

- try indomethacine to facilitate spontaneous closure
- elective surgery at 1-2 years
- operate early if large left to right shunt present

Fallot's Tetralogy

- consider palliative surgery for very small severely cyanotic infants (subclavian artery to pulmonary artery anastomosis)
- total correction: surgical mortality up to 15%

Transposition of the Great Vessels

- newborn: palliative enlargement of atrial septal defect ("pull-through" of balloon catheter)
- anatomic correction at 6 months (high surgical mortality)

RESPIRATORY DISEASES

Respiratory Distress Syndrome

- oxygen supplementation
- intubate and ventilate if in respiratory failure (PEEP)
- intratracheal application of artificial surfactant

SIDS

supine versus prone:
- preterm infants with respiratory distress or infants with gastroesophageal reflux do better sleeping in prone position
- positioning infant on their side or back (supine) reduces risk for SIDS

Cystic Fibrosis

- prognosis usually limited by lung disease (initially Staph. aureus, later Pseudomonas)
- try: chest physical therapy, antibiotics, bronchodilators…

GASTROINTESTINAL DISEASES

Tracheoesophageal Fistula
- elevate head of bed to prevent esophageal reflux into lung
- drainage of blind pouch
- surgical correction
- evaluate for other abnormalities

Pyloric Stenosis
- pyloromyotomy

Intussusception
- fatal if untreated
- barium enema is both diagnostic and therapeutic

Infantile Botulism
- prevention: avoid contaminated food (honey !)
- antitoxin neutralizes circulating but not (irreversibly) bound toxin
- supportive care

Meconium Ileus or Plug
- suspect cystic fibrosis !
- contrast enema may be therapeutic in case of plug
- rectal biopsy if suspicion for Hirschsprung's

Malrotation of small intestine
- high risk of ischemia, perforation and sepsis
- surgery (up to 20% mortality)

Hirschsprung's Disease
- resection of aganglionic segment after 6 months of age
- prognosis significantly poorer if enterocolitis present

GENITOURINARY DISEASES

Polycystic Kidneys
- diagnosis: ultrasound
- monitor renal function
- manage complications of renal failure
- strict blood pressure control
- genetic counseling

Wilm's Tumor
- resection and multi-agent adjuvant chemotherapy
- cure rates up to 90%

Cryptorchidism
- observe: 80% of undescended testes are in the scrotum by age of 1 year
- surgical repair is indicated after puberty
- if uncorrected: failure of spermatogenesis, increased risk for seminoma, but normal androgen production

NEUROLOGICAL DISEASES

Cerebral Palsy
- prevention: improved prenatal care and obstetric management
- spasticity sometimes reduced with diazepam or baclofen

Poliomyelitis
- most cases in the US occur in immunodeficient patients who received live vaccine
- bed rest, fever and pain control
- intubation and assisted ventilation may be necessary

Febrile Seizures
- anticonvulsants (phenobarbital) only for high risk infants with recurrent febrile seizures
- if age of onset < 1 year or duration > 15 min : increased likelihood of future chronic epileptic disorder

Reye's Syndrome
- (encephalopathy with acute fatty liver degeneration)
- supportive treatment, vit. K
- treat increased intracranial pressure: hyperventilation, mannitol infusions, ventricular drainage

Retinoblastoma
- (white pupil reflex)
- enucleation, radiotherapy. Goal: minimize tumor, maximize vision
- adjuvant chemotherapy if optic nerve is involved

<u>METABOLIC DISORDERS</u>

Congenital Adrenal Hyperplasia
- goal: suppression of endogenous ACTH
- lifelong daily oral hydrocortisone:
  increase dose 3 to 5fold during periods of stress (fever, surgery etc.)
- lifelong daily mineralocorticoid if salt wasting:
  does not need to be adjusted for stress

Congenital Hypothyroidism
- primary prevention: iodine supplementation prevents endemic hypothyroidism (cretinism)
- secondary prevention: mandatory screening programs (T4, TSH)
- levothyroxine for maintenance therapy

Wilson's Disease

- (hepatolenticular degeneration)
- lifelong penicillamine for symptomatic and asymptomatic cases
- dietary copper restriction not practical
- daily vit. B6 to prevent optical neuritis

INJURY AND POISONING

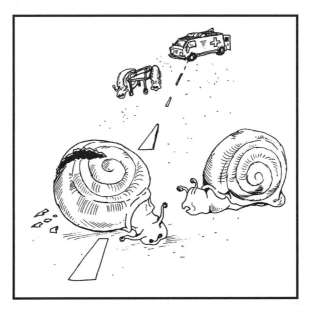

"Easy, John, help will be here any day now."

18.1.) HEAD TRAUMA

concussion	- brief loss of consciousness - no identifiable neuropathological changes - CT scan normal - transient amnesia (anterograde and retrograde)
contusion	- cerebral edema - diffuse intracerebral hemorrhage (coup and contra-coup) - if localized: focal signs - if generalized: focal signs plus impaired mentation
epidural hematoma	**CT: lenticular shape (convex)** - injury of arteries (often middle meningeal artery) - **brief lucid interval**, followed by headache and rapidly decreasing level of consciousness
subdural hematoma	**CT: follows outline of skull (concave)** - injury of bridging veins - **delayed for days or weeks after injury** (occasionally acute) - more common in elderly and alcoholics

basilar skull fractures	- often missed on x-ray
	- watch for signs: **hemotympanum
	                mastoid ecchymosis
	                periorbital ecchymosis
	                facial palsy
	                CSF in nasal sinuses**

 MRI is more sensitive than CT for small hematomas.

18.2.) <u>CHEST TRAUMA</u>

pneumothorax	- spontaneous or following trauma - sudden chest pain - hyperresonance
tension pneumothorax	- sudden chest pain, hyperresonance - ventilatory and circulatory compromise - mediastinal shift - rapidly fatal
open pneumothorax	- from penetrating injury - small wounds may create tension pneumothorax (valvelike mechanism)
hemothorax	- penetrating or blunt trauma - often combined with pneumothorax - shock, hypotension
flail chest	- multiple rib fractures - unstable segment moves inward during inspiration ("paradoxical movement") - respiratory distress
pulmonary contusion	- a/w rib fractures - pulmonary infiltrates on CXR - hypoxemia
cardiac tamponade	- penetrating chest trauma - hypotension - jugular vein distention (unless patient is severely hypovolemic)
aortic dissection	- often fatal - progressive hypotension and shock - mediastinal widening

18.3.) ABDOMINAL TRAUMA

hemorrhage	- injury of: liver, spleen, vessels - *if shock and hypotension are present: assume intraabdominal hemorrhage until excluded by CT, laparoscopy or lavage*
peritonitis	- intestinal injury - pancreatic injury - fever, tachycardia, diffuse pain, ileus
spleen rupture	- **most common injury of blunt abdominal trauma** - left upper quadrant pain - may radiate to shoulder - intraabdominal hemorrhage (shock, hypotension, peritoneal signs) - CT scan is highly sensitive
liver injury	- **most common injury of penetrating abdominal trauma** - right upper quadrant pain - intraabdominal hemorrhage (shock, hypotension, peritoneal signs)
intestinal injury	- usually due to penetrating trauma - small intestinal injury is more common - large intestinal injury is more severe (peritonitis)

Indications for peritoneal lavage:
- *unexplained hypotension and shock*
- *low thoracic penetrating wounds*
- *inability to evaluate abdomen (spinal cord trauma, unconscious patient)*

18.4.) <u>ACUTE ABDOMEN</u>

	if yes consider:
female patient ?	- ruptured ectopic pregnancy - ruptured ovarian cyst - torsion of ovarian tumor
evidence of trauma ?	- perforation - hemorrhage
evidence of obstruction ?	- intussusception - volvulus - incarcerated hernia
evidence of peritonitis ?	- appendicitis - diverticulitis - pancreatitis
hypovolemic shock ?	- ruptured aortic aneurysm
others	- toxins - gastroenteritis - UTI

18.5.) <u>GENITOURINARY TRAUMA</u>

bladder rupture	- common with pelvic fractures - **gross hematuria** (urine sample by catheterization) - acute abdomen indicates intraperitoneal rupture
urethra disruption	- **high prostate** on rectal exam - bloody urethral discharge - may result in impotence and incontinence
kidneys	- common in motor vehicle accidents - degree of hematuria not related to degree of injury - flank pain, lower rib fractures **minor injury** - subcapsular hematomas - contusions **major injury** - vascular injury - deep lacerations - retroperitoneal hemorrhage

18.6.) <u>FRACTURES</u>

hip	- osteoporosis **- avascular necrosis of femur head**
ribs	**- pain that worsens with deep breathing** - flail chest: inward movement during inspiration
Colle's	- breakage and displacement of distal radius **- from fall on outstretched hand**
elbow	- more common in children - watch for injury of median nerve and radial artery **- avoid Volkmann's contracture** (ischemic damage)
pelvis	- most commonly due to motor vehicle accident **- blood loss** !
tibia	**- compartment syndrome:** pain, pulseless, puffy, paresthesia, paralysis
Pott's	- fracture of distal fibula and torn off internal malleolus **- following foot eversion and abduction**

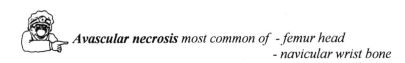

Avascular necrosis most common of - *femur head*
- *navicular wrist bone*

18.7.) <u>NERVE INJURIES</u>

damage to :	results in impaired function of :
axillary nerve	- shoulder abduction
musculocutaneous nerve	- elbow flexion
median nerve	- thumb extension
ulnar nerve	- index finger abduction
femoral nerve	- knee extension
obturator nerve	- hip adduction
superior gluteal nerve	- hip abduction
inferior gluteal nerve	- hip extension
tibial nerve	- foot plantar flexion
peroneal nerve	- foot eversion

18.8.) <u>THE SEA AND THE MOUNTAINS</u>

drowning	- death from fluid aspiration (90%) - or due to laryngospasm (10%) - freshwater (hypotonic) may cause intravascular hemolysis - otherwise little difference to sea water
near-drowning	- pulmonary edema - pneumonitis - adult respiratory distress syndrome - cerebral edema - cardiac arrhythmias
decompression sickness (Caisson disease)	- rapid ascent from deep sea diving - rapid ascent in unpressurized aircraft - symptoms occur **within 30 min to hours** - joint pain - skin mottling - burning, prickling sensation - cough, dyspnea - coma
arterial gas embolism	- rapid ascent from deep diving - symptoms occur **within minutes** - seizures - myocardial infarction
high altitude sickness	- headache, dizziness - nausea, vomiting **pulmonary edema** - resting dyspnea, wheezing or orthopnea **cerebral edema** - ataxia, confusion - papilledema, retinal hemorrhage

18.9.) <u>ANTIDOTES</u>

aspirin	dialysis
acetaminophen	N-acetylcysteine
anticholinergics	physostigmine
organophosphates	atropine, pralidoxime
digitalis	lidocaine antibodies
opiates	naloxone
benzodiazepines	flumazenil
tricyclic antidepressants	sodium bicarbonate
methanol	ethanol
ethylene glycol (anti freeze)	ethanol
CO	O_2
cyanide	amylnitrate
iron	deferoxamine
lead	penicillamine

Hot-List

Head Trauma
- **concussion**: careful observation
- **epidural hematoma**: urgent surgery to avoid brain herniation
- **acute subdural hematoma**: surgery
- **slow subdural hematoma**: this is the "classic" high risk patient who becomes symptomatic days or weeks after the incident

Chest Trauma
- **rib fractures**: analgesia, encourage patient to cough and breath !
- **flail chest**: may require endotracheal intubation, monitor blood gases
- **pneumothorax**: convert tension pneumothorax to open pneumothorax
- **great vessel injury**: emergency thoracostomy

Abdominal Trauma
- penetrating gun shot wounds: surgery
- splenic rupture: splenectomy or repair if possible
- laparotomy if patient has falling hematocrit or blood pressure

Pelvic Trauma
- monitor patient for hemorrhagic shock
- urethral bleeding: obtain urethrogram before inserting a Foley catheter
- microhematuria found by catheter but no shock or pelvic fracture: observe
- cystogram to exclude bladder rupture

Sprains
- rest, ice, compression, elevation
- NSAIDs
- knee joint: early mobilization important

Dislocations
- morphine to reduce pain and allow muscle relaxation
- immediate closed reduction
- **shoulder dislocation**: anterior is easier to fix than posterior dislocation

- **hip dislocation** (usually posterior) often due to motor vehicle accidents. Urgent reduction (probably "open") required to avoid avascular necrosis of femur head

Fractures
- **clavicle**: posterior T-splint
- **humerus**: hanging cast, exercise to prevent stiffening of shoulder. If fracture is distal watch out for Volkmann's ischemic contracture !
- **radius, ulna**: closed (or open) reduction, intraosseus pins
- **wrist**: scaphoid fractures are easily overlooked and are a common site of non-union
- **cervical vertebrae**: if suspected: immobilize immediately
- **pelvis**: 6-8 weeks bed rest
- **femur neck**: common site of non-union. Avoid abduction plaster cast. Better: internal fixation.
- **tibia (±fibula):** plaster splint
- **Pott's**: closed reduction, plaster cast

Drowning
- "the patient isn't dead until he/she is warm and dead"
  (immersion in cold water slows brain metabolism)
- resuscitate immediately
- don't waste time attempting to drain water from victims lungs or stomach
- if patient survives: hospitalize and watch for signs of pneumonitis or pulmonary edema

Decompression sickness
- oxygen
- analgesics
- recompression

Burns

- Rule of 9: head 1, arms 1+1, legs 2+2, front torso 2, back torso 2
- large volume fluid resuscitation (crystalloids). Adjust to maintain urine output > 0.5 ml/kg/h
- expect cardiac arrhythmias (electrolyte imbalances)
- expect ileus if > 20% surface burned

Insect Stings

- rapid onset of urticaria, respiratory distress and hypotension indicate anaphylactic reaction
- epinephrine, antihistamines, intubation

Animal Bites

- danger of infection: **monkey > cat > dog**
- cleanse, debride and irrigate wound
- cephalosporins for cat and dog bites
- hospitalize if infection involves hand
- consider rabies prophylaxis
- **skunks, bats** : Rabies prophylaxis: Duck embryo vaccine plus hyperimmune rabies immune globulins (HRIG) obtained from human volunteers

Spider Bites

- **black widow spider** (abdominal pain, vomiting, shock): Ca-gluconate
- **brown recluse spider** (fever, rash, jaundice, DIC): Steroids. May require total excision of lesion

Poisoning

- gastric lavage is better than to induce vomiting
- do not induce vomiting if patient unconscious
- do not induce vomiting if caustics or hydrocarbons (oils etc.) have been ingested
- next give 50-100 g activated charcoal (except for acetaminophen overdose)
- specific antidotes see above

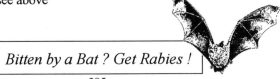

Bitten by a Bat ? Get Rabies !

NEUROLOGY

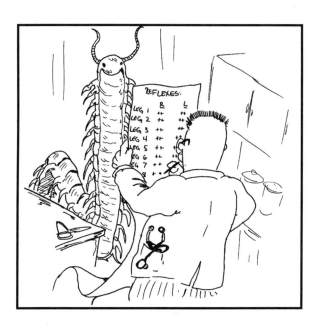

19.1.) <u>CEREBROSPINAL FLUID</u>

	bacterial	viral	fungal	tbc
cells	PMNs	lymphos	lymphos	lymphos
glucose [1]	↓	∅	(↓)	(↓)
protein	↑	∅	(↑)	(↑)

[1] normal is about 2/3 of serum glucose

<u>*Indications for lumbar puncture*</u> *:*
- *suspicion of acute CNS infection*
- *before anticoagulant therapy of stroke if imaging unavailable*

<u>*Contraindications for lumbar puncture*</u> *:*
- *suspicion of brain tumor*
- *increased intracranial pressure*
- *bleeding tendency*

 CSF of newborns*: higher protein content, more lymphocytes.*

19.2.) <u>PUPILS</u>

	light reactive	not light reactive
large	- children - anxiety	- death - atropine poisoning - cocaine, amphetamine
small	- elderly - Horner's syndrome	- Argyll Robertson - opiates

Argyll Robertson pupils respond to near accommodation but do not respond to light.

19.3.) <u>HEADACHE</u>

tension headache	**- steady, nonpulsatile** - unilateral or bilateral
classic migraine	**- preceded by aura** - malaise - nausea - photophobia
common migraine	**- not preceded by aura** - malaise - nausea - photophobia
complicated migraine	**- migraine with neurologic symptoms** that outlast the headache (ischemia): - paresthesias - aphasia
cluster headache	**- severe, unilateral, orbital pain** - occurs in clusters lasting weeks - conjunctiva injection - eyelid edema - lacrimation
tumor headache	**- develops slowly** with increased intracranial pressure - initially mild, occurs after waking up - exacerbated by coughing, bending or sudden movements
meningitis	**- severe throbbing pain**
subarachnoid hemorrhage	**- sudden onset** headache "worst ever"

19.4.) <u>VERTIGO</u>

physiologic vertigo	**- mismatch between vestibular, visual and somatosensory input** - motion sickness - height vertigo - astronauts
brainstem ischemia / tumors	**- vertigo** **- diplopia** **- nausea, vomiting** - occipital headaches
Méniére's	**- abrupt, severe vertigo** **- fluctuating hearing loss** **- tinnitus** - usually unilateral
labyrinthitis	**- abrupt, severe vertigo** - patient unable to sit or stand - nystagmus: away from involved labyrinth

---

> ***Other causes of "dizziness" that might be confused with vertigo:***
> *- ataxia (cerebellar disease or loss of proprioception)*
> *- syncope*
> *- anxiety*
> *- partial complex seizures*

19.5.) <u>SYNCOPE</u>

vasovagal	- due to stress or pain - preceded by nausea, pallor, sweating
cardiac	**- tachyarrhythmias** - preceded by dizziness, palpitations **- outflow obstruction** (cardiomyopathy, aortic stenosis etc.) precipitated by exertion
TIA	- transient focal signs
seizures	- aura - tongue biting - incontinence - postictal confusion
hypoglycemia	- preceded by confusion, jitteriness, tachycardia

 "Coma-Cocktail": give **thiamine, glucose, naloxone.**

19.6.) <u>STROKE</u>

TIA	- <u>transient</u> focal neurologic deficits - lasts minutes to hours - no residual effect
ischemic	**- embolic or thrombotic occlusion** <u>risk factors:</u> - arteriosclerosis - atrial fibrillation - heart valves (septic or non-septic)
hemorrhagic	**- subarachnoid or intracerebral** <u>risk factors:</u> - intracranial aneurysms - arteriovenous malformations - hypertension

hemorrhagic stroke needs to be ruled out before beginning treatment of ischemic stroke !

middle cerebral artery	- contralateral hemiparesis - aphasia
anterior cerebral artery	- contralateral foot and distal leg paresis
vertebral and basilar artery	- amnesia, diplopia, ataxia - visual field defects
lacunar stroke **(small branches of Willis' circle)**	- pure **motor** hemiparesis : internal capsule - pure **sensory** stroke : ventrolateral thalamus - dysarthria, **clumsy** hand : base of pons

A young woman with stroke: think 1.) oral contraceptives
2.) SLE

303

19.7.) <u>CORTICAL SIGNS</u>

frontal lobe	parietal lobe
- contralateral UMN lesion (spastic paresis)	- contralateral impairment of somatesthetic recognition
- aphasia if dominant hemisphere	- aphasia - apraxia } if dominant hemisphere - acalculia
- personality changes	- spatial disorientation - inappropriate affect

19.8.) <u>APHASIA</u>

Broca's	**- inferior frontal gyrus** - nonfluent speech - good comprehension - self aware, frustrated patient
Wernicke's	**- posterior superior temporal lobe** - fluent but nonsensical speech - poor comprehension - often no insight
global	**- large frontal-temporal lesions** - defects in both expression and comprehension

Don't confuse Broca's aphasia with dysarthria (inability to articulate properly due to a motor disorder).

19.9.) <u>TREMOR</u>

physiological	- 8 to 12 Hz - distal extremities
Parkinson's	- 4 to 7 Hz - **resting tremor** - "pill rolling"
cerebellar	- 3 to 6 Hz - **intention tremor** - increases when target is approached
asterixis	- 1 to 3 Hz - **wrist joint flapping**

19.10.) <u>EPILEPSY</u>

generalized seizures (involves both hemispheres)	**nonconvulsive** - absence spells (petit mal) [1] - myoclonic seizures **convulsive** tonic-clonic (grand mal)

partial seizures	**simple**
	(normal consciousness)
	- motor (Jacksonian)
	- sensory (auditory, olfactory...)
	- autonomic (pallor, flushing...)
	
	complex [2]
	(impaired consciousness)
	- most frequent form of chronic epilepsy
	
	- origin in temporal lobe or limbic area
	
	- aura: déja vu
	        foul odor
	        pleasure, fear, anger
	        lip smacking

[1] no aura, no warning, no cataplexy, no postictal period.
[2] most frequent form of chronic epilepsy

 Partial seizures often progress to secondarily generalized seizures.

> *<u>Narcolepsy</u> : <u>REM onset sleep:</u>*
> *- involuntary daytime sleep*
> *- cataplexy*
> *- hypnagogic hallucinations*

19.11.) <u>EEG PATTERNS</u>

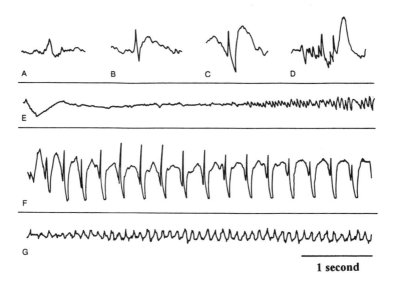

From *Cecil Textbook of Medicine*, 19th edition, p. 2208, edited by J.B. Wyngaarden et al.
Copyright 1992 by W.B. Saunders Co., Philadelphia, PA. Used with permission.

A:	interictal sharp wave
B:	interictal spike-and-wave complex
C:	interictal spike-and-wave complex
D:	interictal polyspike-and-wave complex
E:	onset of generalized convulsion
F:	3/sec spike-and-wave complex (petit mal)
G:	temporal lobe seizure

19.12.) <u>MENINGITIS</u>

neonates (< 1 month)	1. **Streptococci** 2. E. coli 3. Listeria
children (1 month ~ 15 years)	1. **Hemophilus influenzae** 2. Meningococcus 3. Pneumococcus
adults (>15 years)	1. **Pneumococcus** 2. Meningococcus 3. Hemophilus influenzae

Pneumococcus	- penicillin - ampicillin - ceftriaxone
Meningococcus	- same as for pneumococcus **prophylaxis:** - rifampin - tetravalent vaccine (ages >2 years)
Listeria	- penicillin - ampicillin
Hemophilus	- cefotaxime

19.13.) <u>MOTOR NEURON LESIONS</u>

upper motor neuron	lower motor neuron
- spastic paralysis	- flaccid paralysis - fibrillations - fasciculations - atrophy
- increased tendon reflexes - Babinski reflex present	- reflexes decreased or absent

<u>*Fibrillations*</u>:
   - *spontaneous twitching of single denervated*
      muscle fibers due to ACH hypersensitivity
   - *can not be seen through skin*

<u>*Fasciculations*</u>:
   - *spontaneous twitching of motor units*
   - *can be seen through skin*

19.14.) SPINAL CORD SIGNS

Brown-Séquard (trauma, tumors)	<u>ipsilateral</u> - spastic hemiparesis - loss of position and vibration <u>contralateral</u> - loss of pain and temperature
anterior cord (occlusion of anterior spinal artery)	**- spastic paresis** **- loss of pain and temperature** - intact position and vibration
posterolateral cord (syphilis, MS)	**- ataxia** **- loss of position and vibration** - intact pain and temperature
syringomyelia (often congenital)	<u>**lower neck, shoulders, arms, hands**</u> **- loss of pain and temperature** **- wasting of muscles** - intact pain and temperature
Guillain-Barré (acute postinfectious polyneuropathy)	**- motor paralysis**: bilateral, ascending, flaccid **- sensory deficit**

19.15.) <u>PERIPHERAL NEUROPATHIES</u>

hereditary	- Charcot-Marie-Tooth - Friedreich's ataxia - leukodystrophies
toxins	- lead - arsenic - mercury - many drugs
nutritional	- vit. B6 deficiency - vit. B12 deficiency - vit. E deficiency
other acquired	- Guillain-Barré syndrome - amyotrophic lateral sclerosis - diabetes mellitus

19.16.) <u>SLEEP DISORDERS</u>

insomnia	- difficulty initiating sleep - difficulty maintaining sleep - exclude medical conditions - exclude mental disorders such as anxiety or major depressive disorder
hypersomnia	- prolonged sleep - daytime sleep - exclude insomnia, medical and mental conditions
narcolepsy	- REM onset sleep - cataplexy: sudden loss of muscle tone - hypnagogic hallucinations: at sleep onset - hypnopompic hallucinations: at awakening - sleep paralysis (upon awakening)
respiratory	- obstructive sleep apnea - central sleep apnea

$\mathcal{H}ot\text{-}\mathcal{L}ist$

HEADACHE

Tension Headache
- simple analgesics
- relaxation techniques

Migraine and Cluster Headache
- ergotamine plus caffeine for acute attack (as early as possible !)
- prophylaxis may be indicated if > 2 attacks per month: β-blockers, ergot alkaloids

Trigeminal neuralgia
- carbamazepine works well !
- if refractory: add baclofen

CEREBROVASCULAR

TIA
- CT scan to exclude hemorrhage
- anticoagulation
- carotid endarterectomy if stenosis >70% and relatively little atherosclerosis elsewhere in the cerebrovascular circulation

Stroke
- CT scan to exclude intracerebral hematoma
- anticoagulation if stroke is progressing. If stroke is complete it may be prudent to wait 2 days and exclude hemorrhage before beginning anticoagulation.
- corticosteroids may help to reduce cerebral edema
- prognosis: generally better for ischemic infarction (especially lacunar) than hemorrhagic infarction

Intracranial Aneurysm

- bed rest, non-opiate pain relief
- surgical clipping as soon as possible after onset
- overall poor prognosis

SEIZURES

Grand Mal

- many persons have a single seizure with no recurrence. Long term treatment after first attack only if a defined cause can be found.
- monitor drug levels occasionally
- never abruptly discontinue anticonvulsants

Status Epilepticus

- assure airways, IV line
- glucose infusion
- diazepam IV
- if convulsions persist, increase dose or add phenobarbital
- if convulsions still persist: anesthesia, neuromuscular blockade

Petit Mal

- half of children with petit mal will develop clonic-tonic seizures before age 20
- ethosuximide, valproic acid
- IV diazepam for status epilepticus

Narcolepsia

- avoid heavy meals (especially when taking the USMLE exam)
- drugs: pemoline, methylphenidate (Ritalin)

Sleep Apnea

- sleep study to distinguish obstructive from central apnea
- obstructive: weight reduction, continuous positive airway pressure
- central: protriptyline

DEGENERATIVE DISORDERS

Parkinson's
- **early stage**: anticholinergics, amantadine
- later: gradually increasing carbidopa/levodopa as tolerated (dyskinesias)
- **late stage**: when response to levodopa diminishes ("on/off" phenomenon) add anticholinergics or bromocriptine

Alzheimer's
- search for and correct treatable factors contributing to cognitive impairment (depression, endocrine disturbances, multi-drug use, nutritional deficiencies...)
- tacrine is useful in early stages
- advance directive should be drafted as early as possible

Huntington's
- phenothiazines or haloperidol to control dyskinesias
- reserpine to deplete central monoamine stores may be useful
- genetic counseling for offspring (specific test for the gene defect is available)

Multiple Sclerosis
- corticosteroids hasten recovery from acute relapse
- consider immunosuppressive therapy for progressive active MS
- baclofen or dantrolene to improve spasticity
- β-interferone is a promising possibility for relapsing-remitting MS

Guillain-Barré
- exclude porphyria and toxic neuropathies
- early plasmapheresis is very useful
- avoid prednisone (will delay recovery)
- 80-90% will recover completely

316

PSYCHIATRY

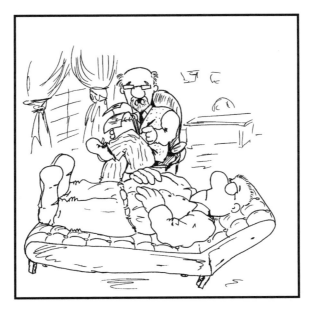

"And how long have you been, in my opinion, evil?"

20.1.) <u>GENETIC FACTORS</u>

mental retardation	**cause often unknown** - the more severe the mental retardation, the more likely it is due to infections, toxins or trauma (often perinatal) **chromosomal abnormalities** - Fragile X - Prader-Willi - Cri-du-chat - Down
schizophrenia	- **50% monozygotic twin concordance** - 12% if one parent has disorder - 40% if both parents have disorder
major depressive disorder	- **50% monozygotic twin concordance** - genetic component not as strong as for bipolar I disorder
bipolar I disorder	- **50-90% monozygotic twin concordance** - 25% if one parent has disorder - 50% if both parents have disorder

20.2.) <u>DSM IV CLASSIFICATION</u>

Axis I	- **clinical** disorders
Axis II	- **personality** disorders - mental retardation
Axis III	- other **medical** conditions
Axis IV	- social and environmental factors
Axis V	- level of functioning

 DSM IV © 1994 American Psychiatric Association. Definitions and diagnostic criteria have been reproduced from the Diagnostics and Statistical Manual of Mental Disorders, Fourth edition, with permission.

20.3.) <u>INFANCY, CHILDHOOD, ADOLESCENCE - 1</u>

mental retardation	- **IQ < 70** (2 standard deviations below norm) - some functional impairment - onset before 18 years
autistic disorder [1]	- impaired social interaction - impaired communication - stereotypic behavior
Aspberger's disorder	- like autistic disorder **without impairment in language** or cognitive development
Rett's disorder	- normal development first 5 months - then : **decelerated head growth**, loss of previously acquired skills, severe psychomotor retardation
Tourette's disorder	- **motor and vocal** tics - onset before age 18 years - duration at least 1 year

[1] must be distinguished from : - selective mutism
                                 - stereotypic movement disorder

20.4.) <u>INFANCY, CHILDHOOD, ADOLESCENCE - 2</u>

enuresis	- age at least **5 years** - significant distress - exclude drugs, medical conditions
encopresis	- age at least **4 years** - exclude drugs, medical conditions
separation anxiety	- excessive distress when separated from parents, going to school etc. - onset before 18 years - ("early onset" if < 6 years of age)
attention-deficit / hyperactivity	- more common in males - at least for 6 months - at least **2 settings**, e.g. home and school - significant impairment in social or academic functioning - may be predominant **inattentive type** - may be predominant **hyperactive type**

20.5.) <u>PERSONALITY DISORDERS - 1</u>

GENERAL CRITERIA:

- **pattern is inflexible across a broad range of situations**
- pattern of experience and behavior is markedly deviant from cultural norms
- significant distress and impairment of functioning

---

paranoid	- distrusting, suspicious
schizoid	- socially detached - **neither desires nor enjoys close relationships** - indifferent to praise or criticism
schizotypal	- **eccentric behavior** - odd or magical beliefs - unusual perceptions - inappropriate affect

20.6.) <u>PERSONALITY DISORDERS - 2</u>

antisocial	**- disregards for rights of others** - reckless, impulsive, irritable
borderline	**- intense but highly unstable relationships** - identity disturbance - self-damaging behavior, suicidal - paranoid ideations - dissociative symptoms
histrionic	- excessively emotional **- needs to be center of attention**
narcissistic	**- sense of grandiosity and self-importance** - sense of entitlement -> envy - lack of empathy -> arrogant behavior

20.7.) <u>PERSONALITY DISORDERS - 3</u>

obsessive-compulsive	**- sense of perfection that interferes with task completion** - preoccupied with details, rules etc. - unable to discard - unable to delegate - rigid, stubborn
avoidant	- social inhibition **- fear of shame or ridicule** - views self as inferior
dependent	- submissive, clinging behavior - difficulty making decisions without reassurance **- feels helpless**

20.8.) <u>AMNESIA</u>

organic	psychogenic
- remote memory intact	- mixture of recent and remote
- emotional events remembered	- emotional events forgotten
- anterograde and retrograde amnesia	- only retrograde amnesia

20.9.) <u>COGNITIVE DISORDERS</u>

delirium	- disturbance of **consciousness** - disturbance of **cognition** (memory, orientation, language) - **rapid onset**, fluctuating - usually due to medical conditions or drugs
dementia	- no disturbance of consciousness - disturbance of **cognition** (memory, orientation, language) - **gradual onset**

Alzheimer dementia	- **exclude:** Parkinson, Huntington, brain tumor,
	  cerebrovascular diseases, hypothyroidism, vit. B12
	  or folic acid deficiency, HIV infection etc.

vascular dementia	- suggested if dementia plus **focal signs**
amnestic disorder	- significant memory impairment - exclude dementia or delirium - "chronic" if longer than 1 month - usually due to medical condition or trauma

	Dementia	**Depression**
insight	- absent	- present
recall of famous persons	- absent	- present
vegetative signs	- rare	- insomnia - constipation - anorexia

20.10.) <u>SCHIZOPHRENIA HISTORICAL CRITERIA</u>

Emil Kraepelin	- "dementia precox" (cognitive process, early onset)
Eugen Bleuler	- "schizophrenia" - schism between thoughts, emotions and behavior - not split personality !
Bleuler's four A	- Associations (formal disorder of thought) - Affect inappropriateness - Autism - Ambivalence
Kurt Schneider	**first rank symptoms:** - audible thoughts - arguing, discussing or commenting voices - somatic passivity experiences - thought withdrawal - thought broadcasting - delusions

 Occasionally, patients may have schizophrenia without showing any of Kurt Schneider's first rank symptoms.

20.11.) <u>SCHIZOPHRENIA CRITERIA</u>

diagnostic criteria	- duration at least 6 months[1] - active phase at least 1 month (unless treated) - must exclude drugs or medical condition !
positive symptoms	- delusions - hallucinations
negative symptoms	- flat affect - alogia - avolition
subtypes	- paranoid - catatonic - disorganized
good prognostic features	- good premorbid functioning - short prodromal phase - absence of blunted or flat affect

[1] includes prodromal, active and residual phase

- ***schizoid*** *personality disorder is unrelated to schizophrenia.*
- ***schizotypal*** *personality disorder is regarded to be the premorbid personality type of many schizophrenics.*
- *however, most persons with schizotypal personality <u>do not</u> develop schizophrenia.*

 Family with high level of expressed emotions increases the probability of a relapse in a schizophrenic patient.

20.12.) <u>SCHIZOPHRENIFORM</u>

schizophreniform disorder	- like schizophrenia - duration **< 6 months**
brief psychotic disorder	- like schizophrenia - duration **< 1 month**

schizoaffective disorder	- major depressive, manic or mixed episode
	  concurrent with symptoms of schizophrenia
	- **delusions or hallucinations for 2 weeks in**
	  absence of prominent mood symptoms[1]

delusional disorder	- **nonbizarre** delusions[2] - criteria for schizophrenia never been met
substance-induced **psychotic disorder**	- **alcohol, hallucinogens, cocaine, PCP...** - prominent delusions or hallucinations - absence of intact reality testing - does not occur exclusively during the drug induced delirium

[1] if delusions and hallucinations occur only during the depressive (or manic) phase it should be classified as **major depressive disorder (or bipolar disorder) with psychotic features** !

[2] real life situations such as being followed, poisoned, loved and deceived etc.

20.13.) <u>ANTIPSYCHOTICS - SIDE EFFECTS</u>

acute dystonia	**- occurs within hours of medication** **(most common with high potency IM dosage)** - torticollis - jaw dislocation - tongue protrusion - *usually disappears eventually (tolerance)* - *switch to another antipsychotic (thioridazine)* - *give anticholinergics*
akathisia	**- may occur at any time** - feeling of muscular discomfort - relentless movements, sit, stand, sit, stand... - *reduce dosage !*
parkinsonism	**- occurs within weeks to months of treatment** - muscle stiffness - cogwheel rigidity - shuffling, drooling - *usually disappears eventually (tolerance)* - *add anticholinergics for several weeks*
tardive dyskinesia	**- occurs after many months of treatment** - choreoathetosis - tongue protrusion - lateral movements of jaw - *reduce dosage, switch or stop* - *most mild cases eventually remit but more* *severe ones are often irreversible*
malignant syndrome	- high fever, heart rate and blood pressure - muscle rigidity - *immediately discontinue drug !* - *cool patient, give dantrolene and anti-parkinson*

329

20.14.) <u>MOOD DISORDERS - EPISODES</u>

major depressive episode	- depressed mood - diminished interest - weight loss - early morning insomnia - feeling of worthlessness **- do not diagnose this within 2 months of bereavement !**
manic episode	- decreased need for sleep - talkative, flight of ideas - goal directed but very distractible **- marked impairment of social or occupational functioning**
hypomanic episode	- markedly elevated mood - uncharacteristic change in behavior **- not severe enough to impair social or occupational functioning** - duration > 4 days

20.15.) <u>MOOD DISORDERS - ENTITIES</u>

major depressive disorder	- presence of major depressive episode - there has never been a hypomanic, manic or mixed episode - exclude schizophrenia
bipolar I disorder	**- at least one manic episode**
bipolar II disorder	- at least one major depressive episode and at least one hypomanic episode **- there has never been a manic or mixed episode**
dysthymic disorder	- depressed mood **for > 2 years** - but no major depressive episode
cyclothymic disorder	- numerous hypomanic periods - numerous depressive periods, but no major depressive episode **- for > 2 years**

20.16.) <u>ANTIDEPRESSANTS - SIDE EFFECTS</u>

tricyclic antidepressants	**- anticholinergic action** blurred vision, dry mouth, constipation, urinary retention - sedation - ECG: prolonged PQ, depressed ST (contraindicated if AV conduction defect) - may induce a manic episode
MAO inhibitors	- orthostatic hypotension - weight gain, edema **tyramine induced hypertensive crisis** (*avoid beer, wine, cheese, fresh oranges...*)
lithium [1]	**- tremors** - nausea, vomiting, diarrhea - confusion - convulsions - coarse tremors and ataxia are the first sign of toxicity (medical emergency) !

[1] prevents both manic and depressive episodes.

 Never ever combine several antidepressants !

20.17.) ANXIETY DISORDERS - 1

panic attack	- abrupt onset, peak within 10 min. - palpitations, tachycardia - sweating - trembling, shaking - lightheadedness - **derealization** : feeling of unreality of the external world - **depersonalization** : feeling of being detached from oneself - fear of dying
agoraphobia	- anxiety of being in **places were a panic attack might occur** and escape would be impossible or embarrassing
panic disorder	- recurrent panic attacks - persistent concern about have additional attacks result in behavioral change - with or without agoraphobia
specific phobia	- persistent excessive fear - cued by presence or anticipation - **patient recognizes that the fear is unrealistic** !
social phobia	- persistent fear of social or performance situations (unfamiliar people, possible scrutiny by others etc.) - **patient recognizes that the fear is unrealistic** !
obsessive-compulsive disorder	- **obsessions**: recurrent thoughts, impulses, images - **compulsions**: repetitive behaviors - **patient recognized at some point that these are unreasonable**

20.18.) <u>ANXIETY DISORDERS - 2</u>

acute stress disorder	- traumatic event -> intense fear - dissociative symptoms [1] - dreams, illusions, flashbacks - **lasts at least 2 days** - **occurs within 4 weeks of event**
posttraumatic stress disorder	- traumatic event -> intense fear - dissociative symptoms [1] - dreams, illusions, flashbacks - persistent arousal, hypervigilance - **lasts at least 1 month** [2] - **occurs any time after event** [3]
generalized anxiety disorder	- excessive worry (work, school etc.) - restlessness, fatigue - irritability, muscle tension - sleep disturbance - **duration > 6 months**

[1] **dissociative symptoms** : derealization
depersonalization
sense of numbing, detachment
absence of emotional responsiveness

[2] considered "**chronic**" if > 3 months

[3] considered "**delayed**" if onset of symptoms > 6 months after event

20.19.) <u>SOMATOFORM DISORDERS</u>

somatization (Briquet's syndrome)	- sickly for most of life - GI, reproductive, cardiopulmonary, pain etc. - diagnosed, when at least 12 symptoms are present and history of several years.
conversion disorder (hysterical neurosis)	- "pseudoneurological" blindness, paresthesia, paralysis - symptoms begin and end suddenly - often misdiagnosed as "malingering"
hypochondriasis	- unrealistic interpretation of body signs - belief to have serious disease that goes unrecognized by family and physicians
factitious disorder	- intentional feigning of symptoms - **motivation: assume the "sick role"** - external incentives (economic gain, avoiding legal responsibilities etc.) are absent !
malingering	- intentional feigning of symptoms - **motivation: economic gain, avoiding legal responsibilities...**

20.20.) <u>DISSOCIATIVE DISORDERS</u>

dissociative amnesia	- **inability to recall important personal information** - goes beyond forgetfulness
dissociative fugue	- sudden, unexpected travel away from home - **inability to recall one's past** - **assume new identity**
depersonalization	- **feeling like one is in a dream** - feeling detached from oneself - reality testing remains intact during this experience
dissociative identity disorder (multiple personality disorder)	- **two or more distinct personalities** recurrently taking control of person's behavior - inability to recall important personal information

*In order to make a diagnosis of dissociative disorder, other causes of amnesia, fugue or depersonalization such as **trauma, drug abuse, acute stress disorder, posttraumatic stress disorder etc. must be excluded.***

Despite the popular notion to the contrary, multiple personality disorder is completely distinct from schizophrenia.

20.21.) <u>EATING DISORDERS</u>

anorexia nervosa	bulimia
- refusal to maintain weight (>15% below normal) - intense fear of becoming fat - disturbed body image - amenorrhea	- lack of control over eating behavior **- recurrent episodes of binge eating** - persistent concern about body weight - self-induced vomiting - abuse of laxatives,diuretics

ABBREVIATIONS

ACE	angiotensin converting enzyme		LMP	last menstrual period
AFP	alpha-fetoprotein		LSD	lysergic acid diethylamine
AGA	appropriate for gestational age		MAO	monoamine oxidase
ANA	antinuclear antigen		MCH	mean corpuscular hemoglobin
ANCA	antineutrophil cytoplasmic antibody		MCHC	mean corpuscular hemoglobin
ARDS	acute respiratory distress syndrome			concentration
ARF	acute renal failure		MCV	mean corpuscular volume
ASD	atrial septal defect		MI	myocardial infarction
ATN	acute tubular necrosis		MMR	measles-mumps-rubella
BMI	body mass index		MS	multiple sclerosis
CEA	carcinoembryonic antigen		NBT	nitroblue tetrazolium
CHD	coronary heart disease		NIDDM	non-insulin-dependent diabetes mellitus
CHF	congestive heart failure		NSAID	non-steroidal antiinflammatory drug
COPD	chronic obstructive pulmonary disease		PAS	periodic acid Schiff
CRFLX	circumflex coronary artery		PCP	phencyclidine
CSF	cerebrospinal fluid		PDA	patent ductus arteriosus
CXR	chest x-ray		PEEP	positive end-expiratory pressure
DHEA	dihydroepiandrostenedione		PIP	proximal interphalangeal joint
DHT	dihydrotestosterone		PMN	polymorphonuclear leukocyte
DIC	disseminated intravascular coagulation		PPD	purified protein derivative
DIP	distal interphalangeal joint		PSA	prostate specific antigen
DM	diabetes mellitus		PT	prothrombin time
DTP	diphtheria-tetanus-pertussis		PTH	parathormone
DUI	driving under the influence		PTT	partial thromboplastin time
E.M.	electron microscope		RA	rheumatoid arthritis
ECV	extracellular volume		RBBB	right bundle branch block
ENA	extractable nuclear antigen		RBC	red blood cell
ERCP	endoscopic retrograde		RCA	right coronary artery
	cholangiopancreatography		RV	residual volume
ERV	expiratory reserve volume		SGA	small for gestational age
FTA	fluorescent treponemal antibody		SIADH	syndrome of inappropriate ADH
G6PD	glucose-6-phosphate dehydrogenase		SIDS	sudden infant death syndrome
GBM	glomerular basement membrane		SLE	systemic lupus erythematosus
GFR	glomerular filtration rate		SS	systemic sclerosis
GN	glomerulonephritis		STDs	sexually transmitted diseases
hCG	human chorionic gonadotropin		TBG	thyroxin binding globulin
HDL	high density lipoproteins		TC	total cholesterol
HLA	human leukocytic antigen		TG	triglyceride
IBD	inflammatory bowel disease		TIA	transient ischemic attack
IC	inspiratory capacity		TLC	total lung capacity
ITP	idiopathic thrombocytopenic purpura		TTP	thrombotic thrombocytopenic purpura
IUD	intrauterine device		UMN	upper motor neuron
IVF	in vitro fertilization		UTI	urinary tract infection
L.M.	light microscope		VC	vital capacity
LAD	left ascending coronary artery		VDRL	Venereal Disease Research Laboratories
LBBB	left bundle branch block		VIP	vasoactive intestinal peptide
LDL	low density lipoproteins		VLDL	very low density lipoproteins
LES	lower esophageal sphincter		VSD	ventricular septal defect
LGA	large for gestational age		WBC	white blood cell

RAPID LEARNING AND RETENTION THROUGH THE MEDMASTER SERIES:

CLINICAL NEUROANATOMY MADE RIDICULOUSLY SIMPLE, by S. Goldberg
CLINICAL BIOCHEMISTRY MADE RIDICULOUSLY SIMPLE, by S. Goldberg
CLINICAL ANATOMY MADE RIDICULOUSLY SIMPLE, by S. Goldberg
CLINICAL PHYSIOLOGY MADE RIDICULOUSLY SIMPLE, by S. Goldberg
CLINICAL MICROBIOLOGY MADE RIDICULOUSLY SIMPLE, by M. Gladwin and B. Trattler
CLINICAL PHARMACOLOGY MADE RIDICULOUSLY SIMPLE, by J.M. Olson
OPHTHALMOLOGY MADE RIDICULOUSLY SIMPLE, by S. Goldberg
PSYCHIATRY MADE RIDICULOUSLY SIMPLE, by W.V. Good and J. Nelson
CLINICAL PSYCHOPHARMACOLOGY MADE RIDICULOUSLY SIMPLE, by J. Preston and J. Johnson
ACUTE RENAL INSUFFICIENCY MADE RIDICULOUSLY SIMPLE, by C. Rotellar
MEDICAL BOARDS STEP 1 MADE RIDICULOUSLY SIMPLE, by A. Carl
MEDICAL BOARDS STEP 2 MADE RIDICULOUSLY SIMPLE, by A. Carl
BEHAVIORAL MEDICINE MADE RIDICULOUSLY SIMPLE, by F. Seitz and J. Carr
ACID-BASE, FLUIDS, AND ELECTROLYTES MADE RIDICULOUSLY SIMPLE, by R. Preston
THE FOUR-MINUTE NEUROLOGIC EXAM, by S. Goldberg
MEDICAL SPANGLISH, by T. Espinoza-Abrams
THE DIFFICULT PATIENT, by E. Sohr
BEHAVIORAL SCIENCE FOR THE BOREDS, by F.S. Sierles
CLINICAL ANATOMY AND PATHOPHYSIOLOGY FOR THE HEALTH PROFESSIONAL, by J.V. Stewart
THE JONAH PRINCIPLE: THE BASIS FOR HUMAN AND MACHINE CONSCIOUSNESS, by S. Goldberg
NEUROLOGIC LOCALIZATION (MacIntosh computer program), by S. Goldberg
MEDLAB (MacIntosh computer program), by S. Goldberg

Try your bookstore for these. For further information and ordering send for the MedMaster catalog at MedMaster, P.O. Box 640028, Miami FL 33164.

Σ **(1.6)**

Lyte   136 | 107 | 68   114
       4.7 | 24 | 4.7

Columbia

410 - 800 - 6916

410

859 - 1100

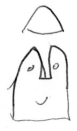